STRABISMUS

A Programmed Text

STRABISMUS

A Programmed Text

second edition

ROBERT D. REINECKE, M.D.

Department of Ophthalmology
Albany Medical College of
Union University
Albany, New York

DAVID MILLER, M.D.

Harvard Medical School
Boston, Massachusetts;
Beth Israel Hospital
Boston, Massachusetts

with a Foreword by Abraham Pollen, M.D.

APPLETON-CENTURY-CROFTS / New York

77 78 79 80 81 / 10 9 8 7 6 5 4 3 2 1

Prentice-Hall International, Inc., London
Prentice-Hall of Australia, Pty. Ltd., Sydney
Prentice-Hall of India Private Limited, New Delhi
Prentice-Hall of Japan, Inc., Tokyo
Prentice-Hall of Southeast Asia (Pte.) Ltd., Singapore
Whitehall Books Ltd., Wellington, New Zealand

Library of Congress Cataloging in Publication Data

Reinecke, Robert D.
Strabismus, Second Edition

Includes index.
1. Strabismus–Programmed instruction. I. Miller, David, 1931- joint author. II. Title. [DNLM: 1. Strabismus–Programmed texts. WW18 R366s]
RE771.R4 1977 617.7'62 77-9539
ISBN 0-8385-8695-3

PRINTED IN THE UNITED STATES OF AMERICA

Contents

Acknowledgments

FIRST EDITION

Psychological Consultant: William Holz, Ph.D.
Medical Illustrator: Jerome T. Glickman
Photographer: Roger C. Lancaster

The research and revision leading to this text was supported in part by U.S. Public Health Research Grant No. NB-05691, from the National Institutes of Health, U.S. Public Health Service, and in part by a grant from the Carnegie Corporation of New York made to the Harvard University Committee on Programmed Instruction.

SECOND EDITION

Medical Illustrators: Ann Veneura and Stephen Shapiro

Portions of the work leading to this second edition were supported by U.S. Public Health Service Research Grant EY-00752 and training grant EY-00044—both from the National Eye Institute and a research grant from Research to Prevent Blindness, Inc.

Preface

The hopes relating to the first edition remain. We believe that the modest amount of additional information contained in this edition should not prove burdensome to the student and should broaden the perspective of care for the strabismic patient. In spite of increasing technology applicable to the quantitation of eye movements, the appropriate treatment includes a strong base of philosophy and "the art" of medicine. If the student attains a measure of how, where, and what to treat, the final product will be well worth our effort as authors and his effort as a student.

Robert D. Reinecke, M.D.
David Miller, M.D.

Preface to the First Edition

Strabismus has been practiced more as an art than as a science. We suspected that a portion of the "art" was composed of predictable facts, and as we delineated the subject this suspicion changed to assurance. Drawing heavily on past studies, we have striven to teach the student those facts which are available. From our tests of this material, students have grasped the concept of strabismus in a satisfactory manner. The student will continue to use the art of medicine in strabismus, but we have noted a slight lifting of the veil of mysticism from strabismus.

The course was tested with the Harvard postgraduate class in ophthalmology. The tests showed revision was necessary, and the appropriate changes were made. We are indebted to the participating students who collectively spent almost one thousand hours taking and critically estimating the course.

We gratefully acknowledge the assistance and cooperation of the Harvard University Committee on Programmed Instruction, Henry F. Allen, M.D., Albert F. Sloane, M.D., The Programming Department of Appleton-Century-Crofts, Anne Chapman, Frances Shapiro, and Billie Louise Young. We give special thanks to David G. Cogan, M.D., Director of the Howe Laboratory of Ophthalmology, where the work was carried out that led to this publication.

Robert D. Reinecke, M.D.
David Miller, M.D.

To the Student

This text is designed to teach you the rudiments of strabismus. Completion of the text should allow you to evaluate critically presentations relating to the subject. Several years of experience are required before you will feel comfortable in your decisions and appraisals of squints, but the text should shorten this period of uncertainty to some extent. The text is not a substitute for clinical experience, nor is it a substitute for practical demonstrations and teaching from your colleagues and peers, but we would hope that the text, used as an adjunct, will give you a firm foundation for other information.

The method of teaching utilized in this text is programmed instruction, and is based upon building a structure of information in a logical fashion. Thus the sequence given should be followed, progressing from frame to frame. Blanks are provided which may be used either to write the response upon, or to be filled in mentally; or you may write the response on another paper. The latter seems the best plan since this keeps the blanks free and the material can be used again. The second time through, the material may be done mentally and should provide a rapid review of the subject.

An index is provided for reference, beginning on page 301.

Prerequisites. This text is written with the assumption that the student has had instruction in refraction. The course–*Refraction*: *A Programmed Text*[1] –may be used to obtain a satisfactory background for this course if the student has had little experience in refraction.

Proceed through the program in the following manner:

1. Read each frame carefully, beginning with frame 1 on page 1.
2. Write your response in the blank or on another slip of paper.
3. Turn to the subsequent frame for the answer.
4. Note that you are to follow the *frame* numbers, not the page numbers. For example, frame 1 is on page 1; frame 2 is on page 3; frame 3 on page 5, etc.
5. After you have completed all the frames in the top layer on the right-hand pages, return to page 1 and continue in the second layer of frames. Go through all the right-hand frames in this way.

6. When you have completed all the frames on the right-hand pages, turn to page 2 and follow the same procedure for the left-hand pages.

7. Occasionally the program will refer you to Table I, page 299, or Panel I, following the index.

We hope you enjoy the course.

[1] Reinecke, Robert D., and Herm, Robert J., *Refraction: A Programmed Text, Second Edition* (New York: Appleton-Century-Crofts, 1976).

Foreword

The rapid expansion of knowledge has resulted in a publication explosion that is beyond the capacity of many to absorb. How to assimilate and digest the ever-enlarging body of accumulated material has posed a challenge for educators in all fields. The authors are therefore to be congratulated on their application of the techniques of programmed learning to the teaching of strabismus. Without attempting to be completely inclusive, the text covers, in a refreshingly unique fashion, the important aspects of the field, ranging from well-established facts to the less well-understood **A-V** syndromes. The emphasis throughout is on the development of the basic science vocabulary and tools so important to the intelligent management of strabismus. It thus prepares the student for the more controversial aspects of theory and the more subtle nuances of differential diagnosis and treatment. For the house officer or recent graduate, it provides a valuable review of essential knowledge and serves as an introduction or supplement to more complicated texts or courses. For the more sophisticated practitioner it affords an interesting and pleasant method of taking stock of one's own knowledge. On all levels, it serves as an excellent adjunct to a more complete understanding of the field of strabismus.

Abraham Pollen, M.D.

PART I BASIC MEASUREMENTS

1. Squint is a condition where both eyes do not look at the same object. A cross-eyed patient (one eye looking at an object, the other eye looking nasally) is said to have a ____________.

149. lower

150. Since a fixation image strikes a point above the fovea of an upward deviating eye, the patient will report this image as being (higher/lower) than the image seen by the fixating eye.

298. higher

299. If a child has an esophoria or esotropia at near which is 10 prism diopters or more greater than the distance measurement, his ACA ratio is greater than 6.

If a child is orthophoric at distance and has a 10 prism diopter esophoria at near, his ACA ratio is considered ____________.

447. (1) left superior rectus } either
(2) right inferior oblique } order

448. The vertically acting muscles are dependent on the horizontally acting muscles. The right inferior rectus can most effectively pull the right eye down when the right ____________ muscle has turned the eye out.

595. exotropia

596. The presence of fusion in most cases of exotropia, as well as in many cases of esotropia, weakens the theory that poor fusion causes squint.

Although poor fusion or no fusion often accompanies squint, why would it be wrong to say that poor fusion causes squint?

743. less (or disappear)

744. Additional plus for near is usually given in the form of bifocals. The wafer bifocals can be cemented on the back of the patient's distance correction.

Additional plus for near is given in the form of ____________.

1. squint

2. Another term for squint is strabismus. A patient who is cross-eyed or wall-eyed (one eye turning out) is said to have a (1) ____________ or (2) ____________.

150. lower

151. The Maddox rod is turned to the vertical position so a horizontal line will be seen, and the vertical phoria is measured with revolving prisms. If the Maddox rod is in front of OD, and the patient sees Figure *A*, the image strikes the lower part of the right retina, and it is projected above the left image. He has a ____________ hyperphoria.

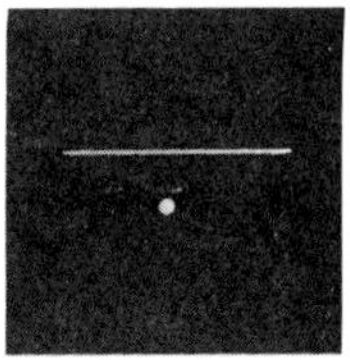

A

299. high (or greater than 6)

300. If a child, whose eyes are always straight, has a high ACA ratio, he does not overconverge when accommodating because his excessive accommodative convergence is neutralized by fusional divergence.

A high ACA ratio can be neutralized by ____________.

448. lateral rectus

449. The obliques can only function as elevators and depressors when the (1) ____________ muscle has turned the eye (2) ____________.

596. Some squinters have good fusion.

597. Present laboratory methods of testing show that the fusional process is probably not present before age six months. Any clinical tests for fusion of a patient prior to age 12 months are difficult and ____________.

744. bifocals (wafer-type bifocals)

745. After an accommodative esotrope has been successfully treated with plus lenses, gradual reduction in the plus over several years can usually be done. An accommodative esotrope of +3.00 D might be expected to (never/eventually) be straight without glasses.

2. (1) squint } either order
(2) strabismus }

3. Besides the terms squint and strabismus, tropia is the technical term (t.t.) used to denote a deviating eye. The prefixes *eso*tropia, for cross-eyes, and *exo*tropia, for wall-eyes, are used. A cross-eyed patient has (1) __________ (t.t.) and a wall-eyed patient has (2) __________ (t.t.).

---

151. left

152. A patient reports the Maddox rod image seen by a hyperphoric eye to be (1) (higher/lower) than the image of the fixating eye. The hyperphoric eye requires prism base- (2) __________ to align the images.

---

300. fusional divergence

301. Fusional convergence or divergence is a process normally used to get a target on corresponding points of each retina when noncorresponding retinal points are stimulated.

If the eyes overconverge for a target, __________ points on each retina are stimulated.

449. (1) medial rectus
(2) in

450. Hering's law states that innervation to yoke muscles is equal. When a patient looks to the right, the right lateral rectus and the left medial rectus receive equal innervation. This last statement is an illustration of ____________ law.

---

597. of no clinical value (or similar words)

598. Since almost 50% of all squints have their onset before age 12 months, when fusion is probably not normally fully developed, it is difficult to implicate poor fusion as a cause of squint.

Why is it difficult to implicate poor fusional development as a cause of squint?

---

745. eventually

746. Plus lenses correct accommodative esotropia by dissociating the amount of accommodative convergence used for any one distance. Plus lenses dissociate the ____________ for any one distance.

3. (1) esotropia
(2) exotropia

4. A patient may say he has a **cast** to his eye. This usually means the patient has a squint but does not imply the type. The **cast** may be either (1) ____________ (t.t.) or (2) ____________ (t.t.).

152. (1) lower
(2) down

153. If the patient has a Maddox rod over OD and sees figure *A*, he has a right hyperphoria. This is measured and corrected with prism base- (up/down) OD. (Remember that a prism moves an image toward its apex.)

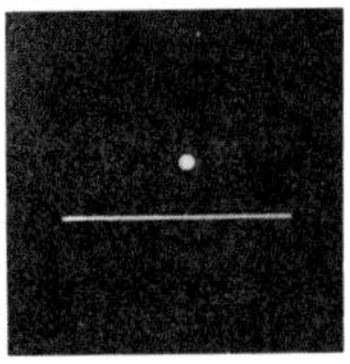

A

301. noncorresponding

302. If a child is looking at the TV and his mother enters the room from the side door, the child's attention is drawn to the door, and his eyes turn to his mother. The chances are that with one quick sweep, the image of his mother will not fall on corresponding points of both retinas. The fusional process will then make a quick correction of eye alignment so that the image of the mother stimulates corresponding points.

Overshoot of the eye(s) is corrected by the ____________ process.

450. Hering's

451. Hering's law implies that when the eyes are looking down and to the left, the right superior oblique muscle and the left (1) ____________ muscle receive (2) ____________ innervation.

598. Most squints occur before normal fusion is developed.

599. The argument for defective fusion causing squints is further weakened by finding stereoblind patients who have straight eyes, and that the congenital unilateral blind-eyed patient typically has (straight eyes/esotropia).

746. accommodative convergence

747. Miotics are drugs which constrict the pupil and stimulate accommodation. Miotics can be used instead of plus lenses to change the amount of accommodative convergence used at any one distance. The miotics seem to work by stimulating a bit of accommodation in the eye, though making the brain think accommodation has been maximally stimulated, and hence reducing the accommodative impulses necessary from the brain. Since less innervation is necessary for accommodation, (more/less) innervation will be used for accommodative convergence.

4. (1) esotropia
(2) exotropia } either order

5. *Strabismus* is the Greek term for squint. *Squint* is an old term meaning "to look obliquely or askance with envy." The Greek term meaning "to look obliquely" is ______________.

153. down

154. Heterophorias (or phorias, for short), vertical and horizontal, are measured at 6 meters using a fixation light. The fixation light is simply a small light bulb. At near, a penlight is frequently used. The Maddox rod can be used in both instances.

To measure distant and near phorias (using a Maddox rod and revolving prisms) a ______________ is a suitable fixation point.

302. fusional

303. One might consider a patient with esotropia to have overconverged in looking at a specific target, and then having managed to direct one eye back on the target.

Esotropes may be thought of as ______________ converging and then not being able to realign both eyes through their fusional process.

451. (1) inferior rectus
(2) equal

452. The deviation called secondary deviation is noted when the paretic eye fixates in the field of action of the paretic muscle. This deviation is greater than the deviation noted when the non-paretic eye fixates in the same field of action. The greater deviation noted when the paretic eye fixates is called a ______________.

599. straight eyes

600. It is known that about 10% of all esotropes become straight when their hyperopia is corrected. How does correction of hyperopia alter the position of the eyes in esotropia?

747. less

748. Miotics change the ACA ratio by reducing the necessary accommodation and hence accommodative convergence. The miotics can be said to ______________ the ACA ratio and provide a new, temporary, lower ACA ratio.

5. strabismus

6. The term cast as a synonym for squint is derived from one meaning of cast which is "to turn, twist, or warp." At least three terms which mean an in-turning or out-turning eye are ________.

154. light (fixation light or equivalent)

155. The range of normal for heterophoria measures 0 to 4△ exophoria when the patient is fixating at 6 meters. When the patient fixates at near (1/3 meter) the average is 3 to 6△ exophoria. Although these are the averages, many values well outside these measurements may be considered physiologic for an asymptomatic patient. If a patient were 1△ exophoric at distance and 7△ exophoric at near and asymptomatic, would the horizontal phorias be abnormal?

303. over

304. If a person has inherited the tendency to squint and also has a high ACA ratio, his fusional process may not be able to neutralize both these tendencies, and he may develop an esotropia.

The combination of an inherited squint tendency and a high ACA ratio may produce an ________.

452. secondary deviation

453. Secondary deviation exemplifies Hering's law. Since the paretic eye needs more innervation to force the paretic muscle to move, the same innervation is sent to the yoke muscle in the non-paretic eye. Secondary deviation is an example of ____________ law.

600. By relaxing accommodation, accommodative convergence is inhibited and the eyes straighten (or similar wording).

601. Some investigators feel that squint is caused by an abnormal accommodative influence on the convergence area of the brain.

How could an abnormal ACA ratio cause an esotropia?

748. reduce (change)

749. Long-acting miotics such as Phospholine Iodide* (echothiophate iodide) can be instilled once a day or less and provide maximal dissociation of accommodative convergence so that many accommodative esotropes will be straight (with/without) their glasses.

*Campbell Pharmaceuticals

6. strabismus, squint, cast, tropia (any three in any order)

7. Strabismus is a major pediatric problem occurring in about 3.5% of children, about the same incidence as diabetes in adults. Of 1000 children, how many would be expected to have squint?

155. no

156. **X** is the usual abbreviation for exophoria at distance and **X′** for exophoria at near. The following prisms measured the horizontal phorias.

6△ base-in at distance
2△ base-in at near.

The phorias would be recorded as (1) ________ , (2) ________ .

304. esotropia

305. Distant vision requires almost no convergence to see singly since the interpupillary distance is not significant compared to 20 feet or infinity. We assume the visual axes to be ________ for distant single vision.

453. Hering's

454. Secondary deviation allows the examiner to tell which muscle is paretic. If an esotropia is present only in right lateral gaze and is worse during right eye fixation than during left eye fixation, the right lateral rectus must be paretic. The left medial rectus receives too much innervation when the paretic ______________ muscle is innervated during OD's fixation to the right.

601. Each unit of accommodation bring along an excess of convergence which is not balanced by fusional divergence.

602. Many esotropes are emmetropic or myopic and have normal ACA ratios. In exotropia, there is no predominating refractive error or accommodative anomaly.

Could the faulty accommodation theory account for the cause of all squints?

749. without

750. Long-acting miotics such as echothiophate iodide and DFP (di-isopropyl fluorophosphate) are especially useful in attempts to remove plus lenses.

Long acting miotics can frequently be used to replace ______________.

7. 35

8. Since the coordinating mechanism of the extraocular muscles is a delicate arrangement, any central nervous system disorder will be expected to show a high incidence of squint. Cerebral palsy, mongolism, and mental retardation are all severe central nervous system disorders, thus all have a (low/high) incidence of strabismus.

156. (1) 6△ **X**
(2) 2△ **X′**

157. Esophoria is frequently abbreviated **E** for distance and **E′** for near. Using these abbreviations:

6△ base-out for distance = (1) ________
3△ base-out for near = (2) ________

305. parallel

306. Near single binocular vision requires convergence. The nearer the object of regard, the more convergence necessary. The convergence necessary for an object 20 cm from the nose is (more/less) than that required for an object 50 cm from the nose.

454. right lateral rectus

455. The secondary deviation is a useful sign to help us in deciding which muscle is paretic. The patient who has an esotropia only on left gaze is noted to have a much greater eso when the left eye fixates to the left than when the right eye fixates to the left. This (1) ____________ deviation implies that the (2) ____________ muscle is paretic.

602. no

603. Although most squints may be changed by altering their state of accommodation, it would be wrong to say that a faulty accommodative factor causes squint. Can the accommodative factor be used to change the angle of the squint?

750. plus lenses (or glasses of hyperopes)

751. Echothiophate iodide is usually used in 1/8% to 1/16% concentration starting out with daily applications and gradually reducing the frequency of application.

Echothiophate iodide (1) ____________% is used initially (2) ____________ time(s) a day.

8. high

9. Other conditions which have an increased incidence of strabismus include prematurity at birth, congenital hypothyroidism, toxemia preceding delivery, and being the first or second child as opposed to subsequent births. Premature infants and infants from mothers who had toxemia of pregnancy would be expected to have a(n) (increased/decreased) incidence of strabismus.

---

157. (1) 6△ E
(2) 3△ E′

158. Vertical prisms, 6△ or more, before an eye will dissociate the images so that the horizontal phoria may be measured. For example, to measure a horizontal phoria, a dissociating prism (6△) base-down OD produces the images as in Diagram 1. (*E* is the fixation target.) (The upper *E* is seen by the right eye because of the 6△ base-down OD.) Prism base-__________ is needed to align the *E*'s as in Diagram 2.

(Remember—a prism moves an image toward its apex.)

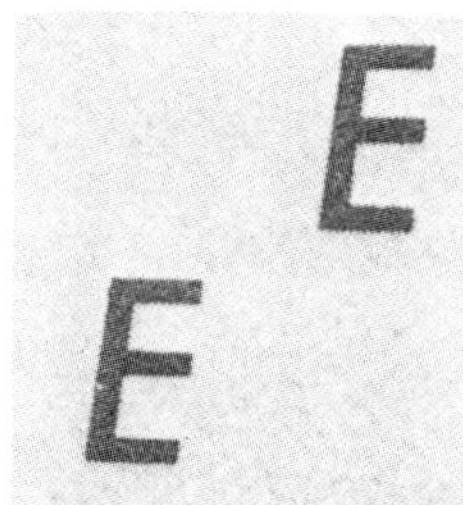

1

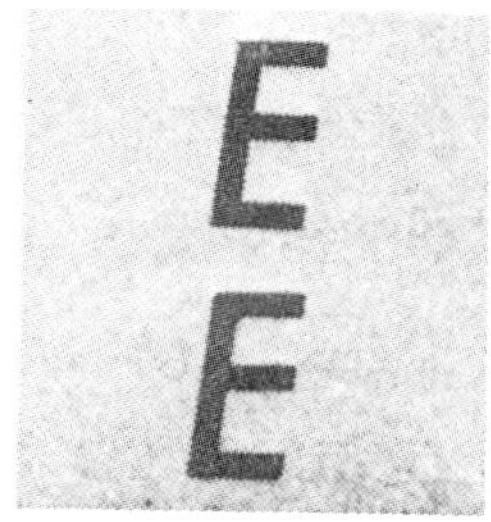

2

---

306. more

307. Focal distances are measured in diopters as 20 cm = 100/20 = 5D. Convergence may similarly be conveniently expressed in its reciprocal. For example, the convergence required to align the visual axes on an object at 25 cm is 100/25 = 4 meter angles. The convergence necessary to align the visual axes on an object at 20 cm is __________ meter angles.

455. (1) secondary
(2) left lateral rectus

456. When there is one weak or paretic muscle in one eye, a noncomitant squint may be present when the eyes are directed to the field of action of the weak muscle. If the normal eye fixates, the paretic eye will simply lag and not quite reach the fixation point. If the paretic eye fixates, there will be extra innervation required for that eye to reach the fixation point. Since Hering's law is valid, the extra innervation will be sent to the yoke muscle of the paretic muscle, and a (larger/smaller) deviation will be noted when the paretic eye fixates than when the normal eye fixates.

---

603. yes

604. The incidence of retinal hemorrhages in normal newborn infants is almost 20%; however, macular hemorrhages are present in only about 2%.

If 100 normal infants were examined during the first day of life, how many would have retinal hemorrhages?

---

751. (1) 1/8 to 1/16
(2) one

752. Echothiophate iodide 1/16% should be refrigerated to prevent deterioration. If Phospholine Iodide is not refrigerated, the beneficial effects on an accommodative esotrope could be expected to ____________.

9. increased

10. Before the age of one year 50% or more of squints become evident; by age four at least 80% of the squints are evident. Most squints develop (early/late) in life.

158. out

159. Dissociation may be produced simply by prisms placed with base perpendicular to the direction in which heterophoria will be measured. For example, to measure a horizontal phoria, 6△ base-down in front of the right eye might produce Figure *A* with the upper *E* being the image seen in the right eye. Additional prism base-__________ would be needed to align the *E*'s so that one is directly above the other and thus measure the horizontal phoria.

A

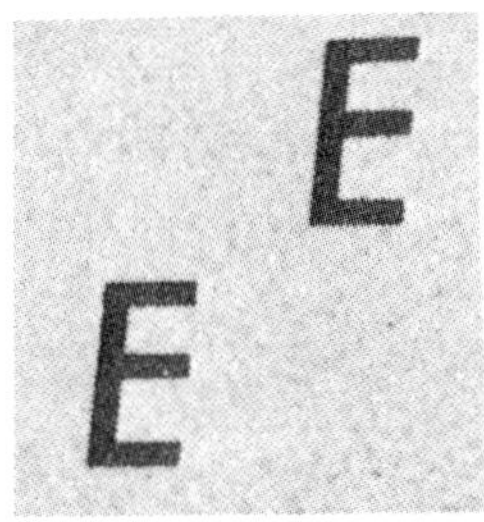

307. 5

308. The number of meter angles is the amount of convergence required to align the (1) __________ on an object. An object at 50 cm will require (2) __________ meter angles of convergence.

456. larger

457. The diagram shows an esotropia which is greatest during OD fixation to the right and illustrates (1) ______ deviation of the left eye. This implies weakness of the (2) ______ muscle.

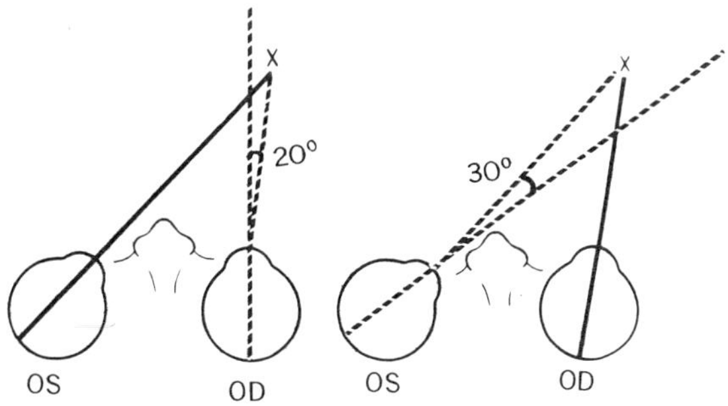

604. 20

605. The large number of retinal hemorrhages following delivery implies that even a normal delivery is traumatic to the eyes.

The common presence of a molded head and black and blue marks on the baby's skin attest to the ______ inherent in the delivery.

752. decrease

753. Di-isopropyl fluorophosphate (DFP) is unstable in water and has to be dissolved in peanut oil. If tears got in a dropper being used to instill DFP, the effect of DFP could be expected to be ______.

10. early

11. Since children sleep a lot, and parents are usually inaccurate observers, the exact onset of a squint is difficult to ascertain. Therefore, the figure of 50% occurrence of squint before age one is probably a(n) (conservative/excessive) estimate.

159. out

160. The vertical phorias are not conveniently measured by utilizing horizontally dissociating prisms because a large amount of prismatic power is frequently necessary to dissociate horizontally.

A better method of measuring vertical phorias is to use the ____________ for dissociation rather than horizontally dissociating prisms.

308. (1) visual axes
(2) two

309. Meter angles indicate only the reciprocal of the distance the object is from the observer. Meter angles do not tell how much an eye must turn in to see singly. To determine how much an eye must converge, the separation of the eyes (PD) must be known. Meter angles (do/do not) indicate the actual convergence required.

457. (1) secondary
(2) right lateral rectus

458. Secondary deviation is an illustration of ________ law.

605. trauma

606. Some theorists believe that during birth one of the nerves going to one of the eye muscles or one of the brain centers controlling the eye muscles may be damaged.

Birth trauma to one of the nerves controlling an eye muscle could produce ____________ of the muscle.

753. reduced

754. DFP is usually used in a concentration of .035%. DFP is unstable in (1) ____________ and the usual concentration of (2) ____________ % would be effectively reduced drastically with only a drop of (3) ____________ .

11. conservative

12. The tendency to squint is inherited as a dominant factor. Other conditions such as high hyperopia, a faulty accommodation-convergence ratio, or a malfunctioning central nervous system determine when and if a squint will become evident.

We (can/cannot) predict the number of children from squinting parents who are affected if we only know whether the parents had strabismus.

---

160. Maddox rod

161. Most patients have a measurable tendency to keep the eyes aligned on one object before they yield to diplopia. This fusional reserve can be measured by utilizing the revolving (variable) prism.

The amount of prismatic power which can be overcome while still maintaining binocular vision is a measure of ____________.

---

309. do not

310. Meter angles is a convenient term, but more information is necessary to determine the amount the eyes turn in. The interpupillary distance (PD) affects the convergence necessary. The greater the PD, the (more/less) convergence will be necessary for a given distance.

458. Hering's

459. An incomitant vertical squint which cannot be explained on the basis of a paralysis or over-action of a muscle is skew deviation. A hypertropia of the right eye in right gaze and the left eye in left gaze may represent a __________ deviation, since there is no muscle abnormality which would cause this deviation.

606. paresis

607. If the muscle that turns the eye out is not working properly, the muscle that turns the eye in works in a more unrestrained manner.

What might happen to the position of the eyes if the lateral recti are weakened and do not equally balance the medial recti?

754. (1) water (or tears) (3) water (or tears)
(2) .035

755. Both DFP and echothiophate iodide cause iris cysts to form. These cysts are prominent along the pupillary border. Patients taking DFP and echothiophate iodide should be frequently examined for the presence of __________.

12. cannot

13. Children who have hyperopia greater than 3.00D have an increased incidence of esotropia. This again indicates that if a tendency to squint is inherited, and a predisposing factor is present, then the patient may be expected to develop a ____________.

---

161. fusional reserve

162. To measure one aspect of fusional reserve, have the patient fixate on a 20/40 letter at 6 meters and increase prism base-in (using revolving prisms) until the patient reports diplopia. Prism base-in is then reduced until single vision is reported. The prismatic powers which result in these two end points are recorded as the break point and recovery point of divergence fusional reserve (or amplitude of divergence) at distance. Divergence fusional reserve is measured with prism base-____________.

---

310. more

311. One prism diopter deflects a ray one centimeter at 100 cm from the prism. A six diopter prism deflects a ray ____________ cm at 100 cm.

459. skew

460. An incomitant vertical squint which cannot be explained on the basis of muscle palsy or overaction is a ______________ deviation.

607. esotropia

608. It is easy to see how the eyes might develop new patterns of movement to compensate for a weakened lateral rectus. Such a pattern might be to always keep the eye turned away from the field of action of the impaired muscle.

If the right eye cannot move to the right, how does the patient utilize his right eye to see what is happening to his right?

755. iris cysts

756. The iris cysts secondary to the use of DFP and echothiophate iodide diminish and disappear as the medicine is reduced or stopped. Phenylephrine used daily with either of the drugs prevents the formation of the cysts. Iris cyst formation can be prevented by (1) ______________ and be reduced if already present by (2) ______________.

13. squint

14. The factors causing an inherited tendency to become an overt squint are multiple. Genetic counseling, in response to parents' inquiry as to future offsprings' likelihood of strabismus, is usually (precise/imprecise).

---

162. in

163. Base-in prism is increased until the break point is reached, and the patient sees double (16△), then it is reduced until he sees singly (8△). This is recorded as divergence fusional reserve 16△/8△.

Divergence fusional reserve 24△/16△ means 24△ base- (1) ______________ caused (2) ______________, and at 16△ base- (3) ______________ he regained (4) ______________.

---

311. 6

312. If a prism deflects a ray 6 cm at 20 cm, the same prism will deflect a ray (1) ______________ cm at 100 cm.

$$\frac{x}{6} = \frac{100}{20}$$

So this prism will be (2) ______________△.

460. skew

461. Skew deviation is a fairly well maintained vertical deviation of the eyes which does not vary in the various fields of gaze appropriate to the extraocular muscle function. The cause is a posterior fossa lesion, but the deviation does not tell where the lesion is located. A vertical squint which varies in the fields of gaze inappropriate to the extraocular muscle function is a (1) ____________ deviation caused by a (2) ____________ lesion.

608. He must turn his head.

609. During birth, a paresis of a muscle which moves the eye up or down may develop. Such a paresis might interfere with the development of binocular movement and eventual fusion. If fusion does not develop, the stage is set for a squint.

How could paresis of a vertically acting eye muscle cause a horizontal squint?

756. (1) concomitant use of phenylephrine or discontinuance of DFP or echothiophate iodide
(2) reduction of DFP or echothiophate iodide

757. Prior to surgery, a thorough eye work-up should be done. For example, a precise visual acuity should be obtained. If vision is low in one eye, the possibility of amblyopia or an organic lesion as a cause should be investigated.

What would be two possible causes of low vision in one eye of a squinting patient aside from a refractive error?

14. imprecise

15. Patient A has (1)__________(t.t.). Patient B has (2)__________(t.t.).

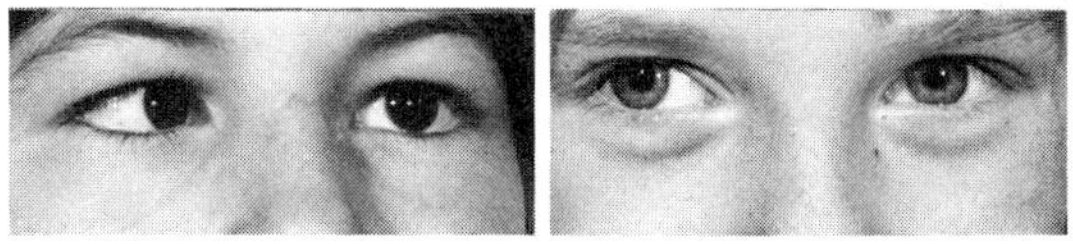

A B

163. (1) in
(2) diplopia (or double vision)
(3) in
(4) fusion (or single vision)

164. Any ametropia except latent hyperopia should be corrected when testing fusional reserves. When divergence reserves at distance are tested, accommodation should play no role, since any relaxation of accommodation will cause an increase in divergence fusional reserves. If accommodation played a role in divergence testing at distance, a patient's lenses did not have enough __________ power.

312. (1) 30
(2) 30

313. If a visual axis (*A-1*) turns in to see *O*, the amount of convergence will be *a*; and *b* will be an amount (equal to/different from) *a*.

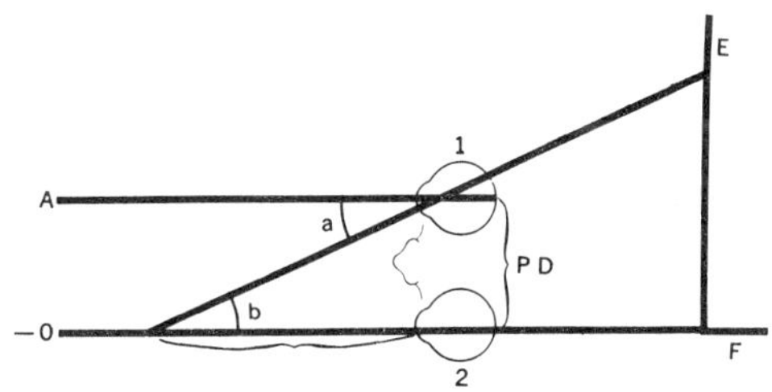

461. (1) skew
(2) posterior fossa

462. Adduction means a movement toward the midline. If the right eye moves to the left (toward the nose), the OD is ____________.

609. Normal development of binocular movement or fusion may be impaired.

610. Once binocular movement is impaired because of paresis of a vertically acting eye muscle in a child, esotropia may develop.

How could the fact that the average young child is about 3 diopters hyperopic account for the development of esotropia if a vertical muscle becomes paralyzed?

757. (1) amblyopia } either
(2) organic lesion } order

758. If no organic lesion is responsible for the low vision, then we are left with an amblyopia due either to anisometropia or a constant squint, or both.

List two causes of amblyopia.

15. (1) esotropia
(2) exotropia

16. The eye muscles are not paralyzed in over 90% of all tropias. The patient shown can move either eye in any direction, indicating that there is no ________.

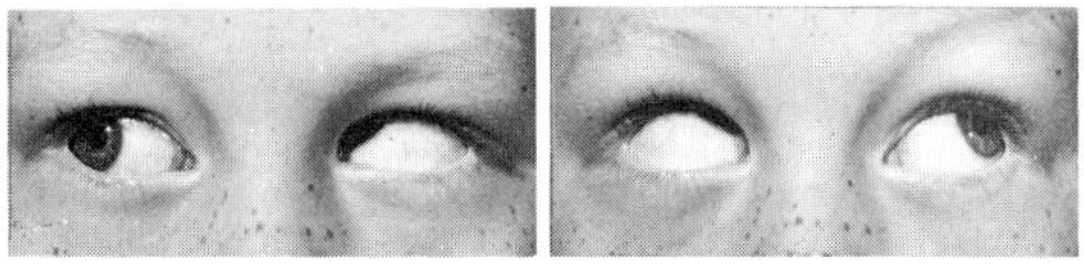

164. plus (or convex)

165. As prism base-in is increased, the eyes must diverge to maintain single vision. The amount of prism base-in which just causes diplopia is a measure of the ________ fusional reserve.

313. equal to

314. Angle b can be expressed in prism diopters and will be that prism which will deflect a ray 6 cm at $33\frac{1}{3}$ cm.

$$\frac{x}{6} = \frac{100}{33\frac{1}{3}}$$

$$x = \_\_\_\_ \quad \Delta$$

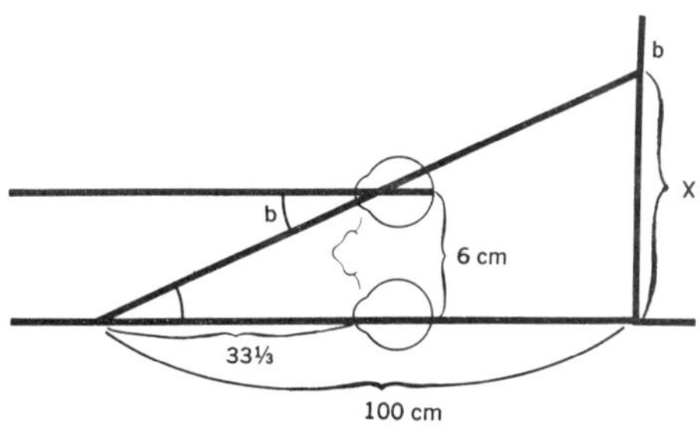

462. adducting (or adducted)

463. Adduction of the right eye means that it moves toward the midline or to the left. Adduction of the left eye means the eye moves to the (right/left).

610. Impaired binocularity and accommodative convergence becoming evident (or equivalent words).

611. A slight weakness of one of the vertically acting muscles has been found in almost 40% of all cases of esotropia.

Of 100 cases of esotropia, how many would also show a weakness of one of the vertically acting muscles?

758. (1) constant squint } either
(2) anisometropia } order

759. A refraction accomplishes two purposes. In a case of amblyopia, it lets you know if a significant anisometropia is present. It also helps determine the amount and significance of the accommodative component in esotropia.

Give two reasons for doing a refraction as part of a squint work-up.

16. paralysis

17. Since patients with nonparalytic tropias have good ocular movements, either eye is capable (with the other eye occluded) of looking in ____________ directions.

165. divergence

166. The amount of prism base-in, which just allows single vision to return after the break point has been determined, indicates the recovery point. The closer the recovery point is to the break point, the greater is the fusional reserve. Which patient has the greatest fusional reserves?

Divergence fusional reserves
(Amplitudes of divergence)

	Diplopia/Recovery
Patient A	16△ B.I./12△ B.I.
Patient B	16△ B.I./ 4△ B.I.

314. 18

315. Six centimeters is the PD, and we see that $\frac{x}{6} = \frac{100}{33\frac{1}{3}}$ gives us the convergence in prism diopters necessary to see an object at $33\frac{1}{3}$ cm. $\frac{100}{33\frac{1}{3}}$ represents the meter angles. So x = PD X ____________.

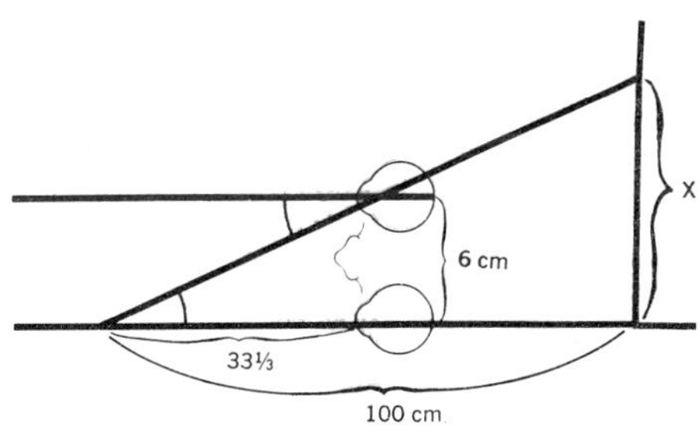

463. right

464. Adduction describes movement toward the midline. Movement away from the midline is termed **abduction**. Abduction of the right eye means OD moves to the (right/left).

611. 40

612. It would appear that congenital vertical muscle palsy may be associated with horizontal squint, but there is no solid proof that it causes horizontal squint. The association may mean that the vertical anomaly has the same etiology as the squint, but cause and effect are difficult to determine. Can you predict that a vertical muscle anomaly will always be present if a horizontal squint is present?

759. (1) determines possibility of anisometropia
(2) determines accommodative component in esotropia
} either order

760. If squint with amblyopia is present, determination of the type of fixation present should be performed with a Visuscope type of instrument.

What instrument helps differentiate central and eccentric fixation?

17. all

18. In nonparalytic squints, the patient cannot align both eyes at the same time but can usually use either eye if the other eye is occluded. Thus if one eye of a patient is covered, you will not know whether the patient has a squint. Can you tell whether the photographed patient has a tropia?

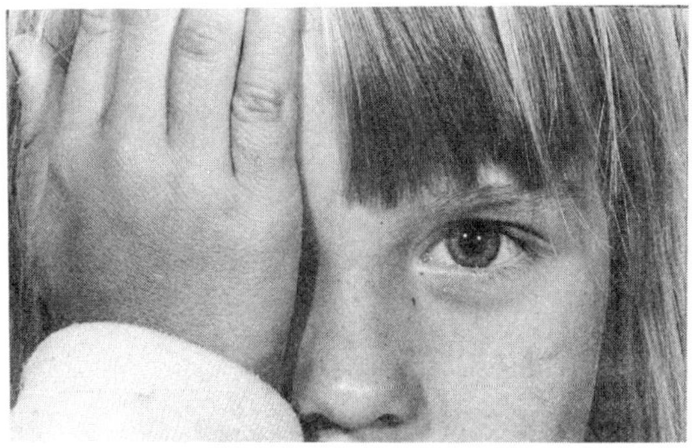

166. A

167. Base-out prisms are used to measure convergence fusional reserve (or amplitude of convergence). Base-out prisms demand that the eyes ____________ to maintain single vision.

315. meter angles

316. The convergence in prism diopters for a given distance equals the product of the PD (in cm) times the ______________ for that distance.

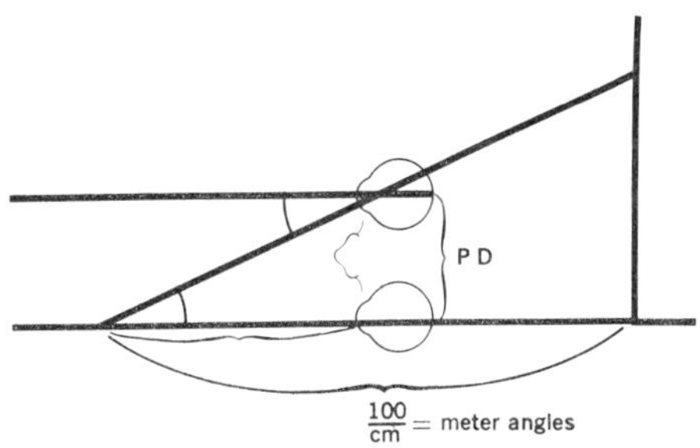

464. right

465. Adduction means a movement toward the midline. Abduction means a movement ____________ the midline.

612. No—also, the vertical problem typically disappears when the horizontal squint is corrected in a child.

613. Plants usually turn their petals toward the light. Some flying insects always turn their bodies toward a light source. These are examples of how light may exert a tonus on the body.

The light is able to turn the insect's body by influencing the ____________ of the insect.

760. Visuscope

761. If amblyopia is present, an attempt to improve vision through an appropriate method should be made before squint surgery.

Should amblyopia treatment come before or after squint surgery?

18. no

19. The patient in the photo has __________ (t.t.).

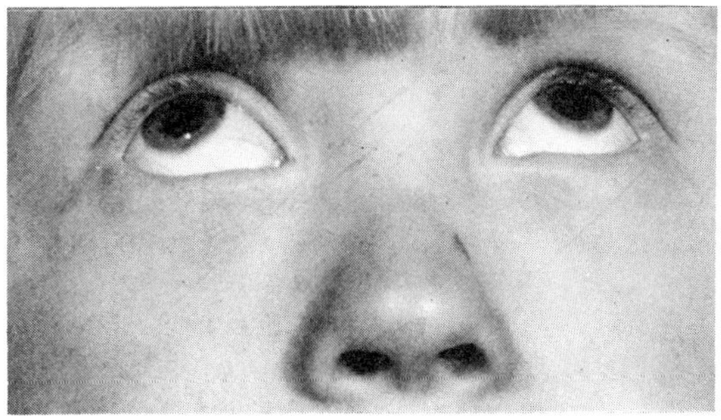

167. converge

168. Convergence and accommodation are closely related. As the eyes accommodate they tend to converge. Esophoria is (greater/less) as accommodation is stimulated.

316. meter angles

317. The prism diopters = PD (in cm) X MA (meter angles). If the PD increases, the convergence required in prism diopters __________.

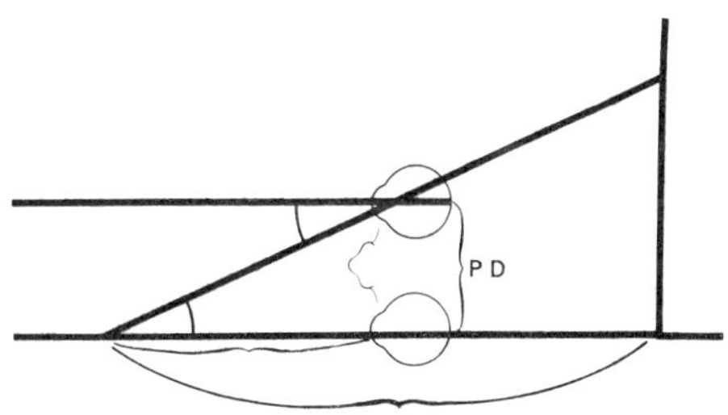

465. away from

466. Abduction means (1) ______________.

Adduction means (2) ______________.

613. tonus (of muscles) (or behavior)

614. In the insect, the light is first picked up by the insect's special light sensors (eyes). Next, a message is sent from the eye to the insect's brain. The brain then directs body movement by sending nerve impulses to muscles.

When we talk of response to light, what important body systems are brought into play?

761. before

762. It has been noted that the likelihood of achieving straight eyes and fusion with surgery is much better if the vision is equal or almost equal in both eyes.

What would be the reason for treating amblyopia before squint surgery?

19. exotropia

20. Can you tell from the photo whether this patient has a squint?

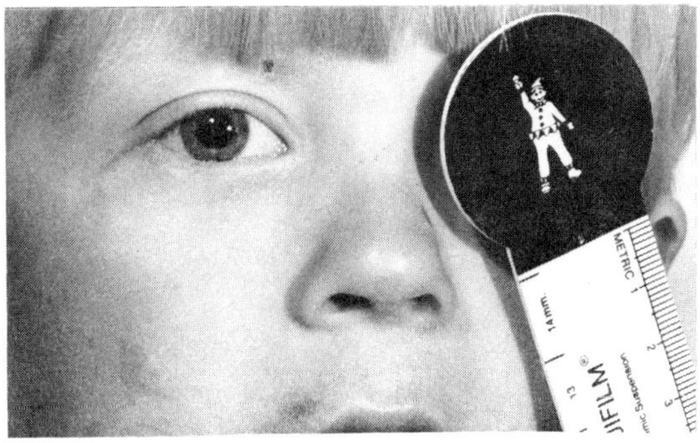

168. greater

169. As prism base-out is increased, the eyes maintain single vision until the convergence reserve is exhausted. Accommodation is then utilized to elicit further convergence to maintain single vision. That convergence, so elicited, is called accommodative convergence (or accommodative fusional reserve). Base-out prisms are increased until the 20/40 line blurs. This is the point at which the patient is beginning to accommodate and thus utilize ____________.

317. increases

318. Δ's = PD × MA.

If the PD is 7 cm, and the distance of the object is 50 cm, the convergence required will be ____________Δ.

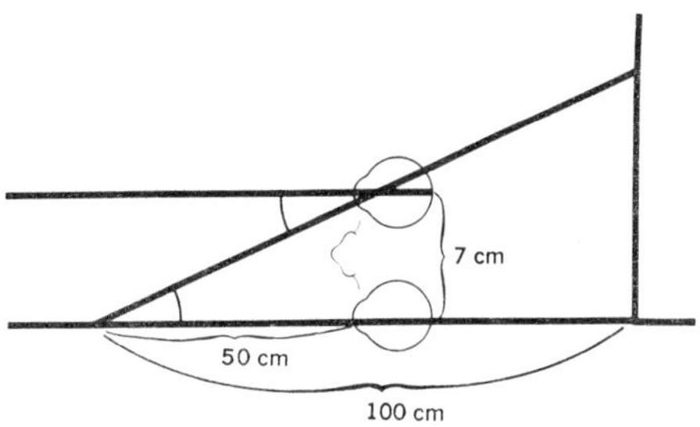

466. (1) movement away from the midline
(2) movement toward the midline

467. Convergence implies that both eyes are rotating toward the midline or ________.

614. eye, brain, nerves, muscles

615. If you were to observe the eyes of a subject as he looks out at the passing scenery from a moving railroad car, you would see them continually jump back and forth in the typical optokinetic nystagmus. A movement of a muscle, elicited by a stimulus and without volition, is called a reflex.

Since the subject is unaware that his eyes are moving and is without volition, the movement is considered ________.

762. The presence of equal or near equal vision in both eyes improves the prognosis.

763. A squint work-up includes a measurement of the angle of squint when fixating at distance and at near. These tests should be done with the patient wearing his proper refractive correction. Squint measurement is done fixating at (1) ________ and at near with the (2) ________ in place.

20. no

21. If you looked behind the occluder, would it be possible to tell whether this patient had a deviated right eye?

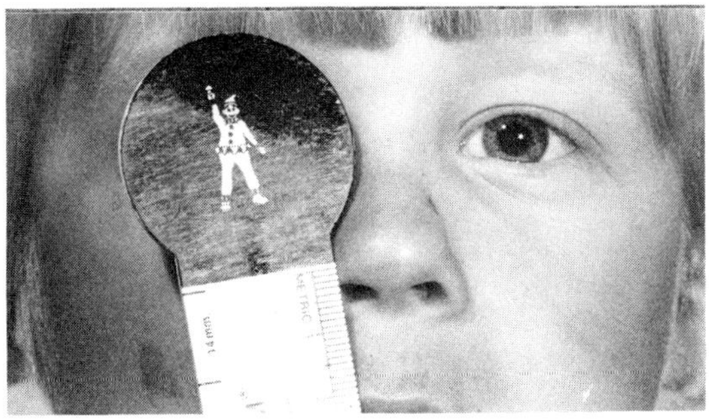

169. accommodative fusional reserve (or accommodative convergence)

170. Base-out prism is increased until the 20/40 line just starts to blur. The amount of this prism is recorded; it measures the convergence (1)____________ at distance. Base-out prism is increased until diplopia is reported. The amount of prism added from the point of blurring until diplopia is reported is a measure of the (2)____________.

318. 14

319. A patient with a PD of 60 (6.0 cm) must converge ____________ Δ to see an object singly at $33\frac{1}{3}$ cm. Δ's = PD $\times$ MA.

467. adducting

468. Both eyes adduct during convergence, but this adduction in convergence is usually called simply convergence. Thus, the adduction associated with a near object of fixation is called __________.

615. a reflex

616. This to and fro reflex movement of the eyes when presented with a moving field of objects is called opticokinetic nystagmus.

What is the eye movement called when a subject is presented with a rotating drum with black and white stripes painted on it?

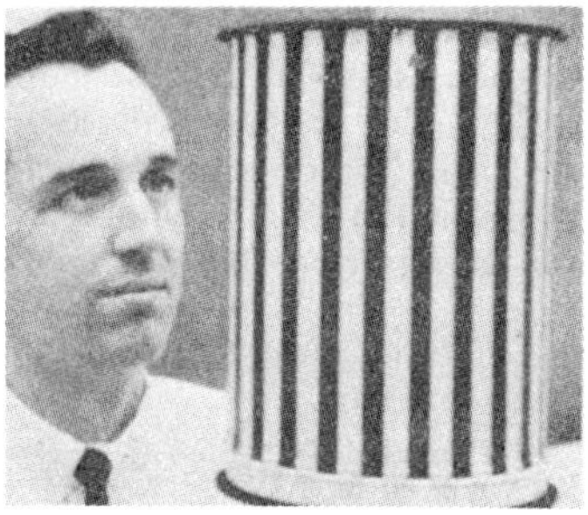

763. (1) distance
(2) refractive correction

764. The accommodative element in esotropia is best picked up by noting either a difference between the near and distance squint measurements or the difference in the size of squint measured with and without glasses.

How would the correction of hyperopia in a case of esotropia with a significant accommodative component affect the angle of squint?

21. yes

22. Photos *A*, *B*, and *C* are of the same patient. Could you tell from *A* or *B* whether the patient had a squint?

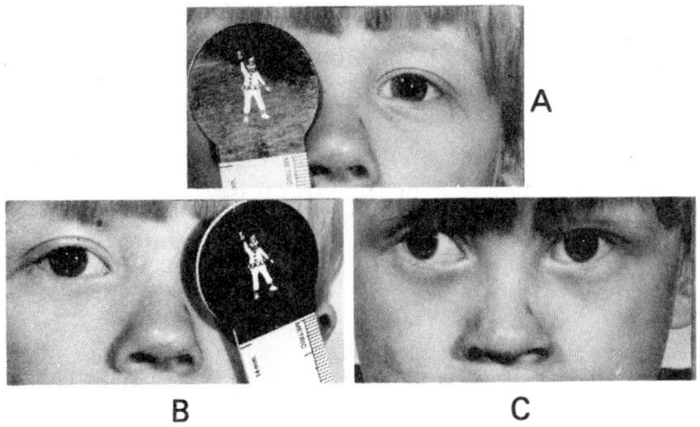

170. (1) fusional reserve (or amplitude)
(2) accommodative fusional reserve (or accommodative convergence)

171. Accommodative fusional reserve is a measure of the accommodation which can be used to stimulate convergence. As accommodation decreases, the accommodative fusional reserve ________ .

319. 18

320. The formula Δ's = PD X MA allows us to calculate the convergence required in prism diopters to see singly, provided the starting position is parallel with the visual axes. If the patient's visual axes are slightly convergent before he attempts to see a near object, the required convergence will be (1) (less/more). If the visual axes are slightly divergent prior to near fixation, the required convergence will be (2) (less/more).

468. convergence

469. The central nervous system (CNS) centers for the control of convergence and for voluntary lateral gaze are separated a short distance but joined by a pathway called the medial longitudinal fasciculus. A lesion in the ____________ may cause a dissociation between the center of convergence and the center for lateral gaze.

616. opticokinetic nystagmus

617. Examples of the effect of light tonus on the eye movements are called **optomotor reflexes.**

Are optomotor reflexes voluntary or involuntary? (1) ____________ . The stimulus for an optomotor reflex depends on the distribution of (2) ____________ on the retina.

764. It would make the squint smaller.

765. In the surgical correction of a partially accommodative esotropia, it is felt that surgery should only attempt to correct the nonaccommodative portion of the squint (ie, the amount present with glasses being worn).

In a case measuring 50△ ET without glasses and 25△ ET with glasses, how much of the squint should be surgically corrected?

22. no

23. The basic squint measurements are done with the patient fixating straight ahead. If measurements are done in other fields of gaze, the amounts may vary in certain circumstances. These circumstances will be covered at a later time. The basic squint measurements are taken with the patient fixating on an object ____________ .
(where)

171. decreases

172. The relation of accommodation to convergence in a given patient may be found by measuring the horizontal phorias before and after stimulating accommodation and noting the phoria change. This is done by having the patient read the 20/40 line wearing his distance correction, dissociating the eyes vertically with 6△ base-up, measuring the horizontal phoria, then placing a −1.00 D sphere OU over his correction and repeating the horizontal phoria measurement. The purpose of the minus 1.00 D sphere is ____________ .

320. (1) less
(2) more

321. The formula for calculating the required convergence in prism diopters is Δ's = (1) ____________ × (2) ____________ .

469. medial longitudinal fasciculus

470. When a patient with internuclear ophthalmoplegia looks to one side, the adducting eye fails to adduct, thus simulating a weakness of the ____________ muscle.

617. (1) involuntary
(2) light

618. If an off-center area of the retina is stimulated by an image, the fixation reflex automatically (involuntarily) rotates the eye so that the image lies on the fovea.

Why is the fixation reflex an optomotor reflex?

765. 25△

766. The squint work-up should include a check for vertical deviation as well as a measure of the horizontal squint with the eyes elevated and then depressed.

A squint work-up should include a search for **A** and (1) ____________ patterns as well as a search for the presence of horizontal and (2) ____________ deviations.

23. straight ahead

24. If a normal eye is looking straight at a target, the rays of light coming from the target are focused on the fovea of the eye.

If we look directly at a target, the image comes to the focus on the ____________ of the eye.

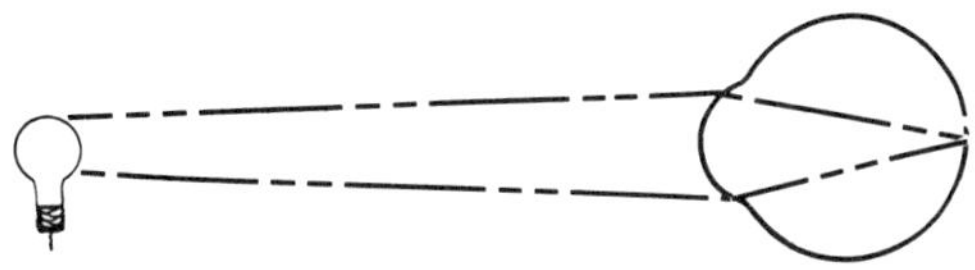

172. stimulation of 1.00 D of accommodation (to see its effect on phorias)

173. The **accommodative convergence/accommodation ratio** (ACA ratio) for a specific individual means that when he accommodates a certain amount, he automatically converges a set amount. One diopter of accommodation for a specific individual will always elicit (the same/variable) amount of convergence.

321. (1) PD (in cm) } either
(2) meter angles } order

322. The patient who has a convergent position of rest while looking at distance (when the eyes are dissociated) will require convergence for near that will be lessened by that amount. If a patient has 4△ esophoria at distance and would require 18△ of convergence if he started with parallelism, he will require only ____________ △ of convergence.

470. medial rectus

471. A rapid to and fro motion of the eye is called nystagmus. There is usually a fast motion in one direction and a slow component in the other direction. ____________ is a rapid to and fro movement of the eyes.

618. An alternation in the pattern of light falling on the retina automatically produces movement (or similar wording).

619. It has been suggested that specific retinal areas may possess specific optomotor values. For example, a point J° left of the fovea when stimulated could incite a J° eye turn to the right. If a retinal area is stimulated 25° to the right of the fovea, the expected eye turn would be (1) ____________° to the (2) ____________ .

766. (1) **V**
(2) vertical

767. If an **A** or **V** pattern of less than 15 prism diopters is present, pure correction of the horizontal squint will usually correct the **A** or **V** pattern. If a patient has a **V** pattern of 10△ ET in the elevated position, he could have up to ____________ △ ET in the depressed position and have only surgical correction of the ET in the horizontal position, since the **V** pattern would be less than 15△.

24. fovea

25. The fovea has the greatest concentration of neural elements capable of discerning fine details. For the best visual acuity, the image of the target must fall on the ____________.

173. the same

174. A 2Δ exophoria at distance might be changed to 1Δ esophoria with a minus 1.00 D sphere OU. This would give an accommodative convergence/accommodation ratio (ACA ratio) of 3Δ/1.00. The ACA ratio of –1.00 D changing a phoria of 2Δ exophoria to 2Δ esophoria would be ____________.

322. 14

323. The patient who has a divergent position of rest will have to actively converge a greater amount to see singly at near. A patient who is 6Δ exophoric will have to converge a total of ____________ Δ to see singly if the convergence required is 18Δ (18Δ starting with parallel visual axes).

471. nystagmus

472. When the patient with internuclear ophthalmoplegia looks to one side, the adducting eye fails to adduct, and the abducting eye shows a nystagmus. As a patient with internuclear ophthalmoplegia looks to the right, the left eye (1) ____________ , and the right eye shows (2) ____________ .

619. (1) 25
(2) left

620. If each retinal area has an optomotor value, then stimulation of the nasal retina would turn the eye out, and stimulation of the temporal retina would turn the eye in.

If point H is stimulated, which way will the eyes rotate to get the image on the fovea? (right or left)

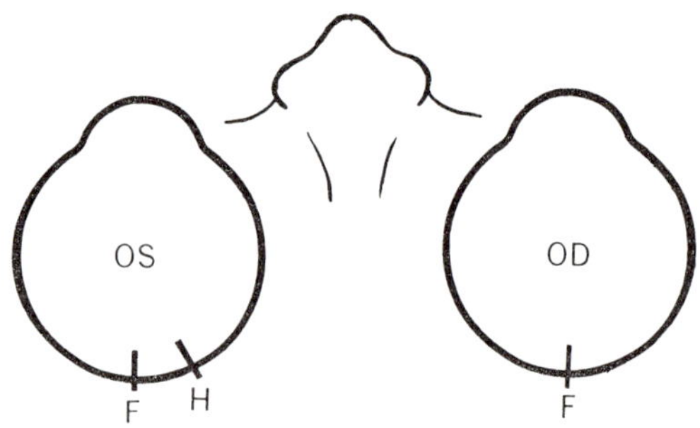

767. 25△

768. A test for abnormal retinal correspondence in a squint work-up helps in deciding the prognosis for fusion after surgery. The presence of ARC makes the likelihood of fusion unlikely.

How does the presence of ARC affect the prognosis of a squint after surgery?

25. fovea

26. Instead of drawing complicated diagrams of light rays coming from an object and being brought to a focus on the fovea, we often just draw a line from the object through the center of the eye to the fovea. This line is called the visual axis. The visual axis is a line connecting the (1) __________ to the (2) __________ .

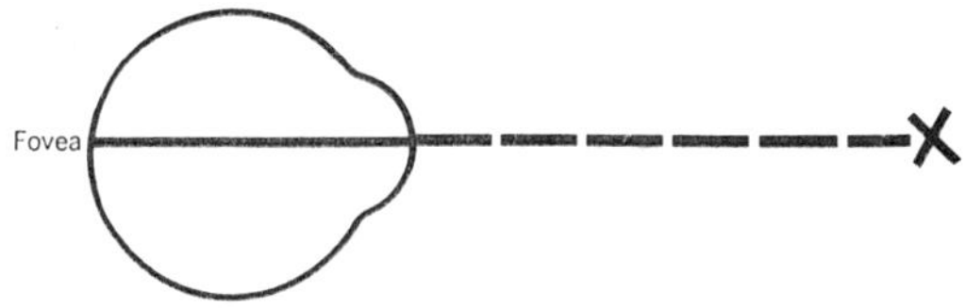

174. 4△/1.00

175. ACA ratio is an abbreviation for __________ __________ .

323. 24

324. The convergence required for any one point is △'s = PD X MA. If the starting position of the visual axes is other than parallel, the active convergence required would be less if the patient were (1) __________ at distance and more if the patient were (2) __________ at distance.

472. (1) fails to adduct (or equivalent terms)
(2) nystagmus

473. A lesion causing damage to the medial longitudinal fasciculus (MLF) may cause the patient to be unable to adduct an eye, thus simulating a medial rectus palsy; yet, the function of the medial rectus can be proven to be intact by having the patient converge and noting the ____________ motion of the affected eye.

620. left

621. It has been shown that the retina nasal to the line through the fovea is anatomically and functionally different from the temporal retina.

If the illustration represents the retina stretched out, and the center dot is the fovea, label the temporal and nasal retinas.

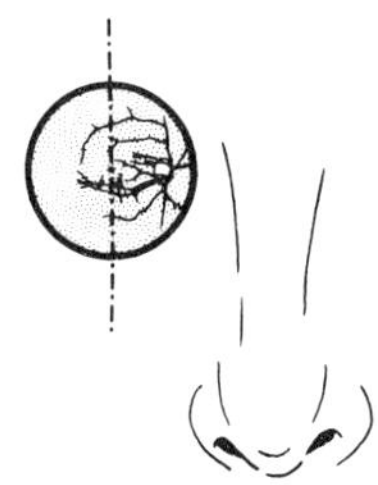

768. makes the likelihood of fusion poor (or equivalent words)

769. The basic principle of squint surgery is to mechanically rotate a turned eye into the straight ahead position. If an eye is turned out, the horizontal muscles are reset in the eye to hold the eye in a straight ahead position.

Would you strengthen or weaken a lateral rectus muscle to correct an XT?

26. (1) target (or object) } either
(2) fovea } order

27. If both eyes in a normal subject are looking at a target, the visual axes of both eyes intersect on the target. An image of *X* is focused on the (1) ____________ of each eye, and the (2) ____________ cross on the target.

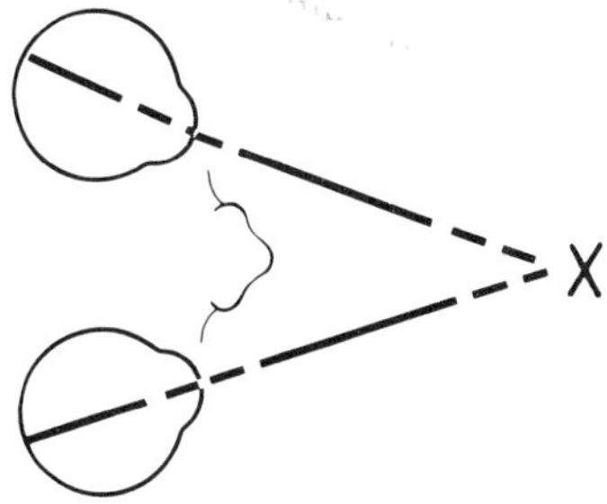

175. accommodative convergence/accommodation ratio

176. If the ACA ratio is large, for example, 6△/1.00, you might expect excessive ____________ at 33⅓ cm (assuming all patients would accommodate the required three diopters for this distance).

324. (1) esophoric
(2) exophoric

325. The ACA ratio allows a prediction of the phoria. An ACA of 6:1 means that the patient will exert 6△ of accommodative convergence for every 1 diopter of accommodation. When viewing an object at 33⅓ cm the patient accommodates 3 diopters and thus exerts ____________ △ accommodative convergence if the ACA ratio is 6:1.

473. inward (or adduction)

474. A lesion in the medial longitudinal fasciculus (MLF) causes an inability to adduct the eye in voluntary gaze to that side, but the function of the medial rectus muscle is proven to be intact by having the patient look at a near object to stimulate ___________ .

621. Temporal | Nasal

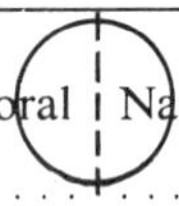

622. The nasal retina has a higher density of rods and cones than the temporal retina, thus there are more cones per square mm on the (nasal/temporal) retina.

769. weaken

770. If the problem of squint surgery were simply to calculate how many degrees the eye must be rotated to assume a straight position, then geometry tells us that every mm on the eyeball is equivalent to about 5°.

In the diagram, if the eye is rotated from point *A* to *B* (a distance of 6 mm), how many degrees does it rotate?

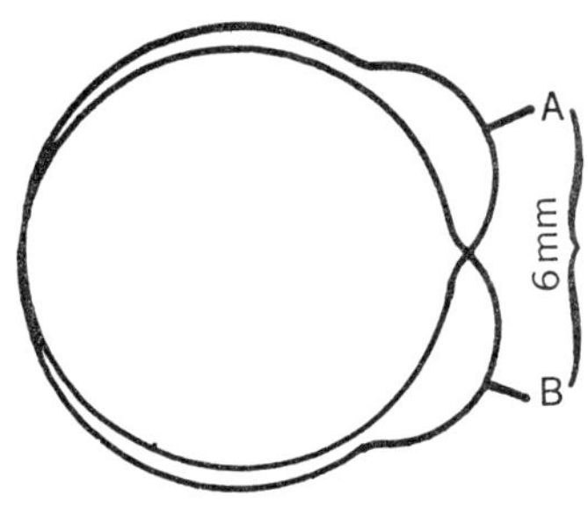

27. (1) fovea
(2) visual axes

28. In the case of a patient with exotropia who is asked to look at a target (*X*), one eye has its visual axis directed to the target, but the other eye's visual axis is directed out. The visual axis of OS (is/is not) directed toward the target *X*.

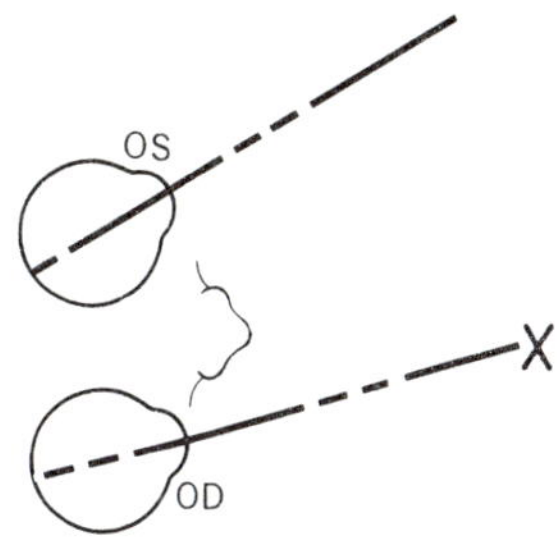

176. convergence (or esophoria)

177. If the ACA ratio is large, a large amplitude of convergence will be found due to the accommodation stimulating relatively large amounts of (1) ____________ and thus maintaining (2) ____________ against more base-out prism.

325. 18

326. An ACA ratio of 4:1 means that ____________ △ accommodative convergence will be used at $33\frac{1}{3}$ cm.

474. convergence

475. An eye which cannot voluntarily adduct, but can use the medial rectus muscle for adduction when converging, is a manifestation of internuclear ophthalmoplegia (internuclear, because the lesion is between the CNS centers or nuclei for (1) ____________ and (2) ____________).

622. nasal

623. The nasal retina is larger in size and comes farther anteriorly than the temporal retina. Does the anterior portion of the nasal or temporal retina lie closer to the cornea?

770. 30°

771. If the average child's eyeball is 22.5 mm in diameter, then the circumference (using the formula, circumference = πd) is about 71 mm. Since there are 360° in a circle, each mm covers about 5°.

If the circumference of a circle were 60 mm, how many degrees would be equivalent to each mm?

28. is not

29. In discussing a case of exotropia, instead of saying that one eye turns out, we may be more precise and say the visual axis of one eye turns out when compared to the other eye.

If the subject in the illustration was asked to look at target *X*, which eye is exotropic?

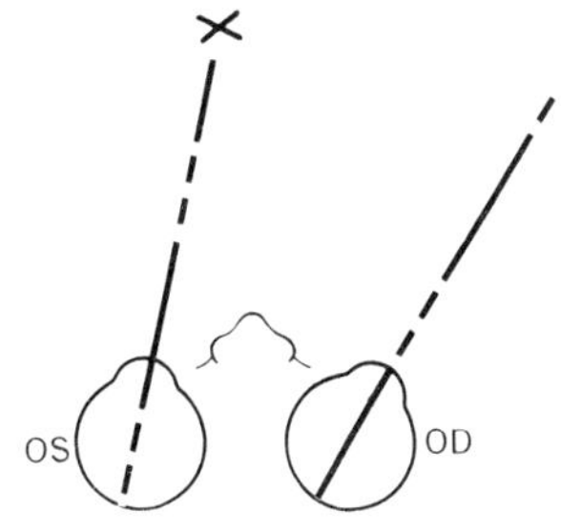

177. (1) convergence
(2) fusion (or single vision)

178. Will the ACA ratio affect the divergence reserves at distance?

326. 12

327. A patient with a PD of 60 (6.0 cm) needs (1) ____________ △ of convergence to see singly at 33⅓ cm. △'s = PD × MA.

The same patient has an ACA ratio of 4:1. This patient will exert (2) ____________ △ accommodative convergence at 33⅓ cm.

475. (1) convergence } either
(2) adduction (or lateral gaze) } order

476. An internuclear ophthalmoplegia is caused by a lesion of the ____________ which connects the CNS centers for convergence and adduction in the brainstem.

623. nasal

624. The nasal retina is older on the evolutionary scale. For example, some fishes who have immobile eyes on the sides of their heads have only a nasal retina.

Name an advantage which eyes on the side of the head have over eyes in front.

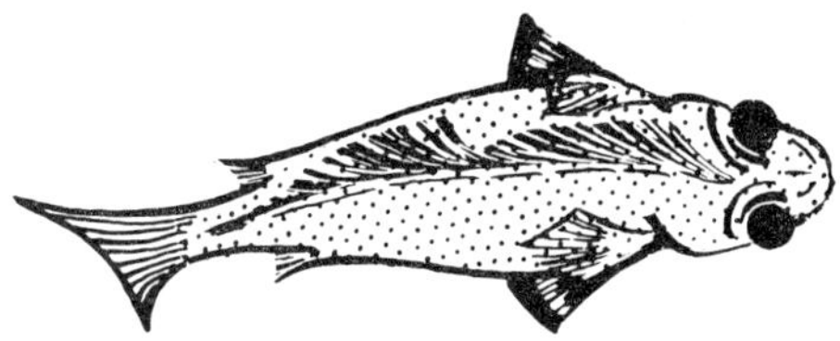

771. 6°

772. The medial rectus and the lateral rectus are the muscles responsible for rotating the eye toward the nose or toward the temple.

The contraction of which muscle rotates the globe nasally?
(1) ____________

The contraction of which muscle rotates the globe temporally?
(2) ____________

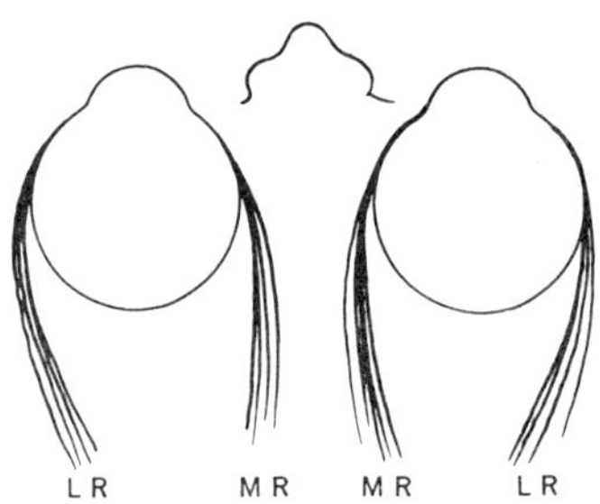

29. OD

30. The visual axis is specific in describing the size of an exotropia. As illustrated, the visual axis of OS is directed toward the target, and the visual axis of OD is directed out. A third line is drawn from the patient's nose to the target. This line helps describe the amount of convergence the fixating eye must turn to look at the target.

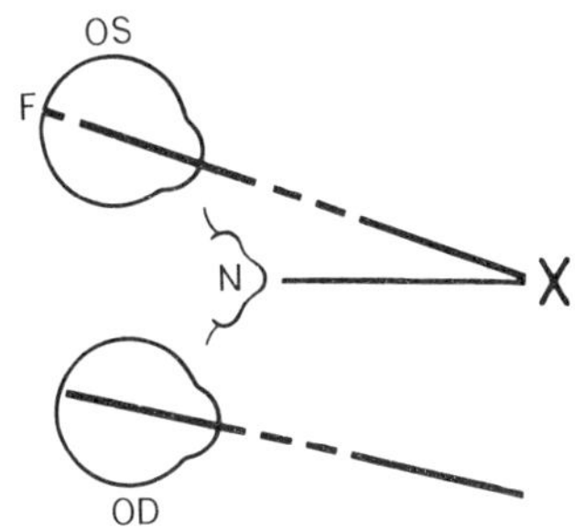

The angle of convergence for the OS is described by the lines (1) ____________ and (2) ____________ .

178. no

179. The ACA ratio affects the divergence reserves at near. If accommodation is relaxed, the accommodative convergence will be reduced, allowing the eyes to diverge, and permitting more base-____________ prism to be overcome at near than at distance with fusion maintained.

327. (1) 18
(2) 12

328. A patient requires 18△ to see singly at 14″ (33⅓ cm), but exerts only 12△ accommodative convergence. If the patient was orthophoric at distance, the near phoria would be an expression of the lack of enough accommodative convergence or ____________ △ exophoria.

476. medial longitudinal fasciculus (MLF)

477. Internuclear ophthalmoplegic patients show nystagmus of the abducting eye. When the patient with internuclear ophthalmoplegia looks to the right, the left medial rectus cannot adduct the left eye to the right, and the right abducting eye shows ____________ .

624. can see in front and beind (or have larger total visual field)

625. If various retinal areas have optomotor values, and if the temporal retina is different from the nasal retina, then the nasal retina may exert a different tonic effect from the temporal retina.

If the temporal retina had a greater combined optomotor value than the nasal retina, which way would the eye turn?

772. (1) medial rectus
(2) lateral rectus

773. In reviewing the anatomy of the medial and lateral recti, we see that they originate from a fixed point in the back of the orbit and attach to the eye at places called the insertions.

Where does the medial rectus originate? (1) ____________

Where does it end? (2) ____________

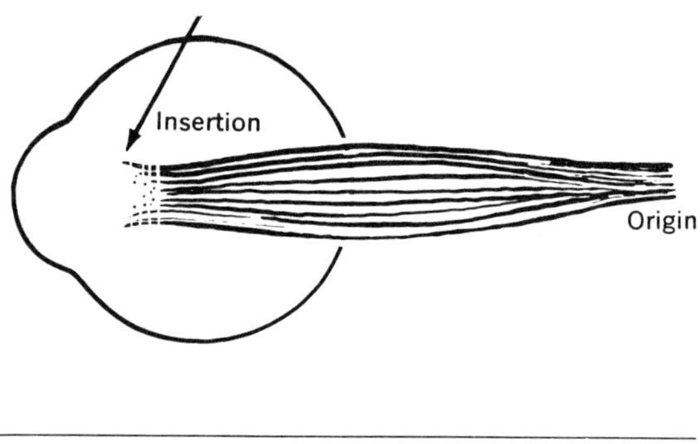

30. (1) FX } either
(2) NX } order

31. Using the same situation, if we draw a line from target X to the right eye and form an angle equal to the one made by lines FX and NX, it will strike the retina of the right eye at a point M.

If the patient in the illustration did not have an exotropia, the visual axis of the right eye would coincide with which line?

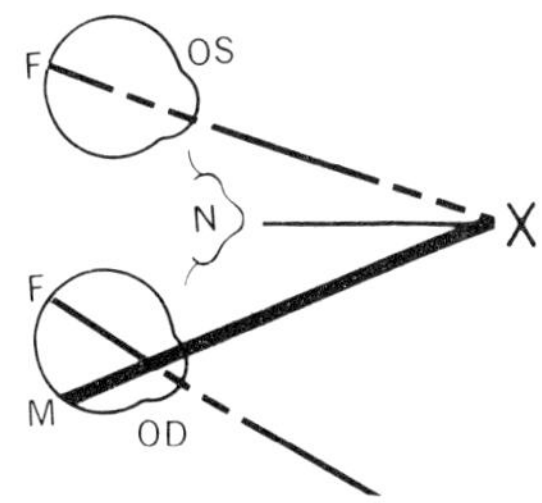

179. in

180. If a patient is orthophoric at distance and 18△ esophoric at near (33⅓ cm), and has an ACA ratio of 6△/1.00, ____________ lenses at near will decrease the accommodation required at near and also decrease the esophoria at near.

328. 6

329. Calculate the following for a single patient:

PD = 70 (7.0 cm); object at 33⅓ cm. Convergence required to see singly is (1) ____________ △ if patient is orthophoric at distance.

ACA = 5:1. Accommodative convergence = (2) ____________ △ at 33⅓ cm. Near phoria = (3) ____________ △ exophoria.

477. nystagmus

478. There are two main causes of internuclear ophthalmoplegia. If the internuclear ophthalmoplegia is bilateral (to both sides of gaze), the lesion is usually due to multiple sclerosis; if it is unilateral (present in gaze only to one side), then the lesion is usually due to a vascular occlusion. The two main causes of internuclear ophthalmoplegia are (1) ____________ and (2) ____________.

625. nasally (medially or in)

626. **Latent nystagmus** is a condition whereby both eyes oscillate to and fro if one eye is covered.

If a patient who has latent nystagmus is looking at something, and one eye is covered, what happens to the uncovered eye?

773. (1) fixed point in back of the orbit
(2) insertion

774. If the lateral rectus muscle is shortened (a piece removed and the ends reattached), the eye would be realigned temporally.

If the lateral rectus is shortened, which way should the eye rotate?

31. *MX*

32. We see that *MX* should be the direction of the right eye's visual axis if there were no exotropia. However, in a case of exotropia, the angle between *MX* and the visual axis is the precise amount the eye is turned out. This is called the angle of squint.

If the angle between *MX* and the visual axis of the right eye is 30°, what is the angle of the squint?

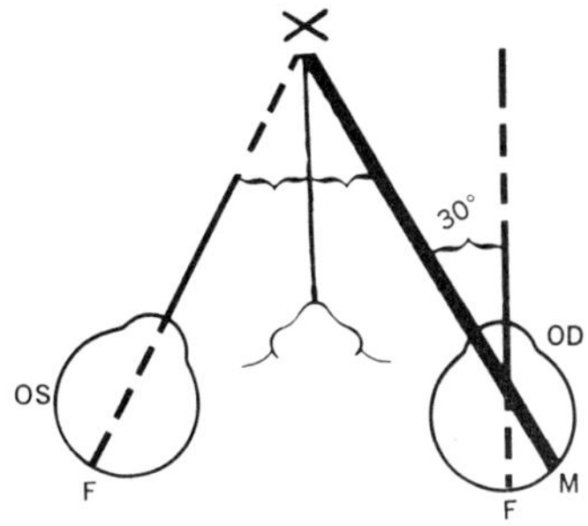

180. plus

181. If the ACA ratio is 6△/1.00, then a +1.50 D add OU at near can be expected to change 12△ esophoria at near to 3△ E′ (esophoria at near). For each 1 diopter of plus, 1 diopter of accommodation is relaxed, and hence 6△ of convergence is abolished. So for 1.50 D of plus, 9△ convergence is abolished, and the phoria changes from 12△ E′ to 3△ E′.

If the ACA ratio is 4△/1.00, then a +2.00 D add OU at near can be expected to change an 18△ esophoria at near to ____________.

329. (1) 21
(2) 15
(3) 6

330. Calculate the following:

PD = 50 (5.0 cm); object at 33⅓ cm. Convergence required to see singly, if patient is 4△ exophoric at distance, is (1) ____________ △.

ACA = 6:1. Accommodative convergence = (2) ____________ △ at 33⅓ cm. Near phoria = ____________ △ exophoria.

478. (1) multiple sclerosis } either
(2) vascular occlusion } order

479. If the internuclear ophthalmoplegia is bilateral, the cause is usually multiple sclerosis; if unilateral, the cause is usually ____________ .

626. It oscillates to and fro (nystagmus occurs equally to both eyes).

627. Some theorists feel that latent nystagmus is due to the uncontrolled tonic imbalance of the nasal and temporal halves of the retina.

How might uncontrolled tonic imbalance of the nasal and temporal retinas cause a to and fro motion of the eyes?

774. temporally

775. When a muscle is shortened by removing a piece of it, the operation is called a resection.

If the lateral rectus is shortened by removing a piece, the operation is called a ____________ of the lateral rectus.

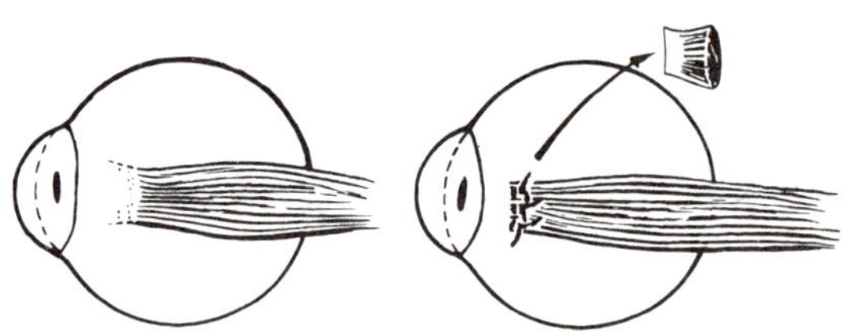

32. 30°

33. In a case of exotropia, the visual axis of the fixating eye makes an angle of 30° with the line from the target to the nose, while the deviating eye looks straight ahead at infinity. Therefore, the deviating eye's visual axis is 30° from where it should be.

The angle of exotropia in this problem is __________.

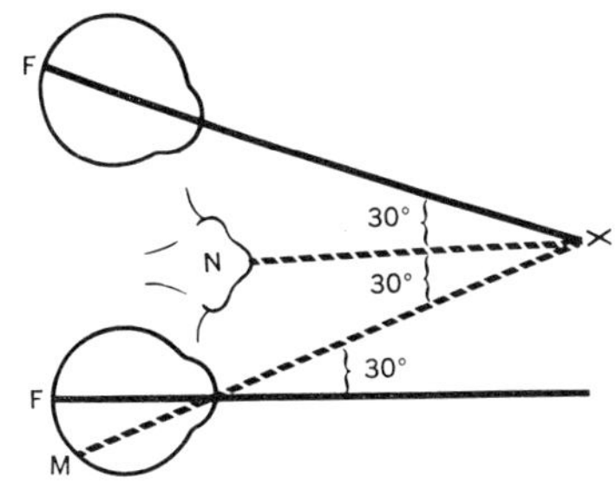

181. 10△ E′ (esophoria at near)

182. Exophoria means the eyes turn (1) __________ when fusion is interrupted; it is measured with prism base- (2) __________ .

330. (1) 19
(2) 18
(3) 1

331. Calculate the following:

PD = 60 (6.0 cm); object at 33⅓ cm. Convergence required to see singly, if patient is 4△ esophoric at distance, is (1) __________ △.

ACA = 6:1. Accommodative convergence = (2) __________ △ at 33⅓ cm. Near phoria = (3) __________ △ esophoria.

479. vascular (occlusion)

480. A moderate divergence or increase in exophoria as the eyes are directed upward is considered physiologic. If the increase in exophoria recorded from looking down 25° to looking up 25° is less than 15△, the difference is within physiologic limits. As the eyes are directed up a moderate increase in ____________ is considered within physiologic limits.

627. A greater nasal tonus might move the eye temporally, then a control would straighten the eye, then the tonic imbalance would exert its force again.

628. Although not a common condition, latent nystagmus is seen more frequently in patients who also have a squint. What group of patients would show a higher incidence of latent nystagmus than the general population?

775. resection

776. A muscle can also be shortened by making a fold in it. This operation is called tucking.

If the lateral rectus is shortened by suturing a fold in it, the lateral rectus is said to have been ____________ .

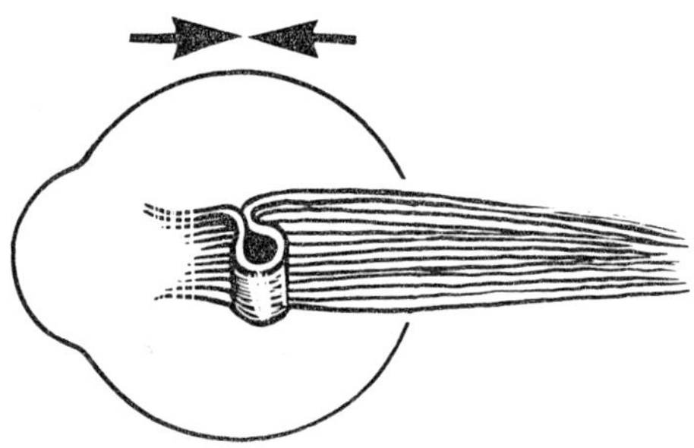

33. 30°

34. In another case of exotropia, the fixating eye is looking straight ahead at a distant target, and the visual axis of the deviating eye makes an angle of 40° with MX. The angle of squint is 40°.

MX in the diagram is the direction of the ____________ if the eye did not deviate.

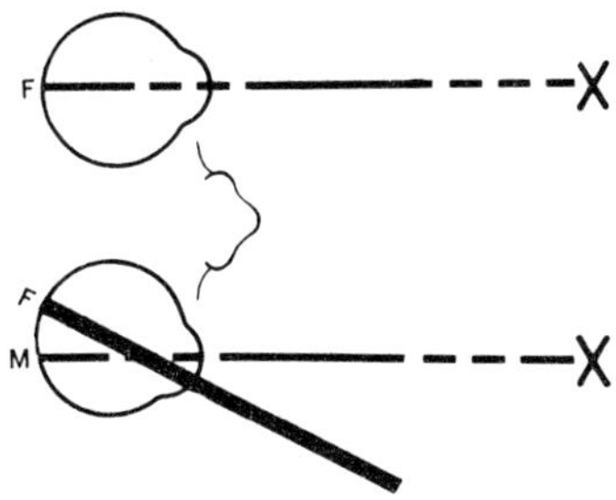

182. (1) out
(2) in

183. Esophoria means the eyes turn (1) ____________ when fusion is interrupted; it is measured with prism base- (2) ____________ .

331. (1) 14
(2) 18
(3) 4

332. Calculate the following:

PD = 60; object at $33\frac{1}{3}$ cm.
Distant phoria = 2△ exophoria.
ACA = 4:1.
Near phoria at $33\frac{1}{3}$ cm = ____________ .

480. exophoria (divergence)

481. If the exophoria increases (or esophoria decreases) more than 15$^{\Delta}$ in changing the gaze from 25° down to 25° up, the pattern of divergence is called a **V** pattern. The **V** means that the eyes tend to diverge more in ____________ gaze.

628. squints

629. Some theorists feel that if a tonic imbalance between retinal halves exists and it is not properly controlled by other reflexes, a squint may result.

Since it is difficult to measure the tonic activity of the two halves of the retina, particularly in young patients, this theory is ____________ .

776. tucked

777. An eye can also be rotated surgically by weakening the pull of a muscle. In essence, this allows the opposite muscle to pull more effectively. If the medial rectus is weakened, which way will the eye rotate?

34. visual axis

35. To review, we describe the angle of the squint by describing the angle (in the deviating eye) between the visual axis and the line *MX*. The direction of the line *MX* is obtained from the visual axis of the fixating eye, or more precisely *MX* is a line from the target through the pupil of the deviating eye.

If the visual axis of the fixating eye points straight ahead to infinity, the direction of *MX* is (1) ____________ , and if the visual axis of the fixating eye makes a certain angle with a line from the nose to the target, the line *MX* makes the (2) ____________ angle with the line from the nose to the target.

---

183. (1) in
(2) out

184. Crossed diplopia (after dissociation) indicates a patient has ____________ .

---

332. 8△ exophoria

333. Calculate the following:

PD = 50; ACA = 6:1; object $33\frac{1}{3}$ cm.
Distant phoria = 2△ esophoria.
Near phoria is ____________ .

481. upward

482. If, instead of diverging when the eyes are directed from 25° down to 25° up, the eyes converge, then the convergence in upward gaze is termed an **A** pattern. An **A** pattern means the eyes ____________ on upward as compared to downward gaze.

---

629. difficult to prove or disprove

630. An eye muscle is considered abnormal if its adhesions to the eye or to the other muscles look excessive or if the muscle is inelastic.

How might a heavy ligament attached from the muscle to the wall of the orbit affect the contraction of the muscle?

---

777. laterally (or temporally)

778. When a muscle insertion is moved back surgically, the operation is called a recession.

If a muscle insertion is moved back, the muscle is said to have been ____________.

35. (1) straight ahead
(2) same

36. You might think that measuring the angle of a squint requires extensive arithmetic. This is not true because of one simple fact. In almost all squint cases, if the fixating eye is covered, the deviating eye moves to pick up fixation.

In the diagram, if a cover is placed before OS (the fixating eye), the visual axis of the right eye will direct itself to ____________.

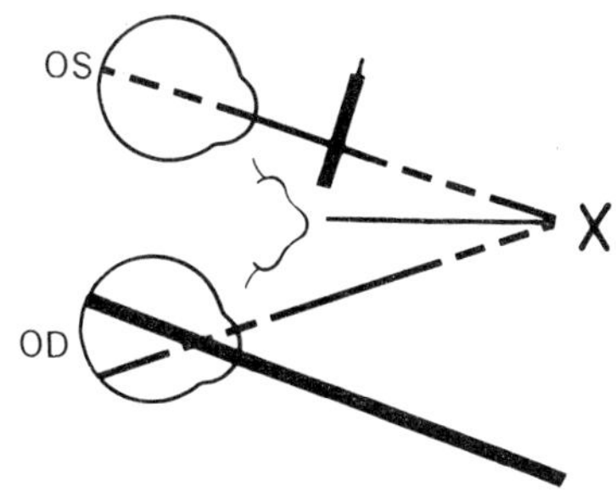

184. exophoria

185. Uncrossed diplopia (after dissociation) indicates a patient has ____________.

333. 5△ esophoria

334. A nonsquinting child with an ACA ratio of 4 and a hyperopia of 4 diopters will have 16 prism diopters of accommodative convergence when looking at infinity.

A nonsquinting child with an ACA ratio of 3 and a hyperopia of 5 diopters will have ____________ prism diopters of accommodative convergence when looking at infinity.

482. converge

483. An **A** pattern means the eyes are more (1) ____________ on upward gaze, while a **V** pattern means the eyes are more convergent on (2) ____________ gaze.

630. A heavy check ligament might interfere with full contraction of the muscle.

631. The diagnosis of an abnormal muscle is usually made during a squint operation.

The diagnosis of an abnormal muscle is made by actually ____________ the muscle.

778. recessed

779. If the insertion of the medial rectus is moved farther back on the eyeball, or recessed, the muscle becomes less taut, or more slack, and is weakened.

What operation makes an eye muscle more slack?

36. *X*

37. When a patient with exotropia looks directly ahead at a distant object, one eye will deviate temporally. If the fixating eye is then occluded, the deviated eye will then look at the object, and the other eye will deviate (temporally/nasally).

185. esophoria

186. Near phorias are measured at 33⅓ cm in the same manner as distance phorias. Dissociation of the eyes is necessary, followed by the use of prisms (preferably revolving) to align the images. Near phorias are measured at ____________ .

334. 15

335. If a child with hyperopia of 4.00 D looks at a target 33⅓ cm away, he must accommodate a total of 7 diopters to see the target clearly.

If a child with a hyperopia of 5.00 D looks at a target 33⅓ cm away, he must accommodate a total of ____________ diopters to see the target clearly.

483. (1) convergent
(2) downward

484. **A** and **V** patterns refer to the relative convergence and divergence in the up and down positions. The eyes may be esotropic in the down position and be more esotropic in the up position, hence be an **A** pattern esotrope. An exotrope may be more exotropic in the up position than the down position and thus be a(n) ____________ pattern exotrope.

631. seeing (or examining or operating)

632. Some investigators have found a high incidence of abnormal-looking muscles in cases of squint. Do esotropes often have abnormal-looking eye muscles?

779. recession

780. The four rectus muscles of each eye (superior rectus, inferior rectus, lateral rectus, medial rectus) are all connected to each other by the intermuscular membrane which circles the posterior portion of the globe.

The ____________ connects all four rectus muscles around the posterior portion of the globe.

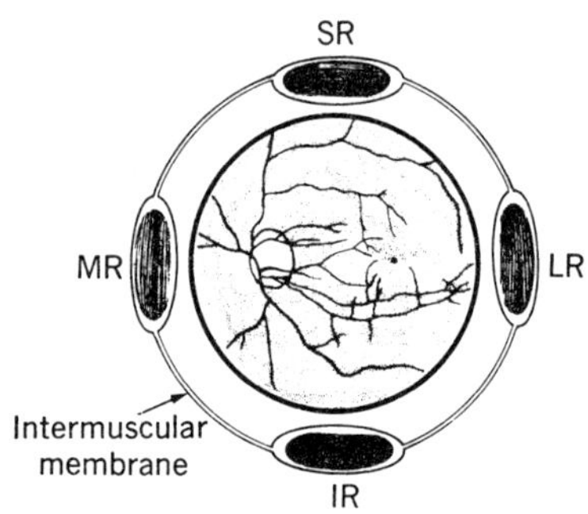

37. temporally

38. As we have seen in the case of exotropia, when the fixating eye is covered, the deviated eye must turn to get the image of the target focused on its fovea. If by some trick the image of the target would fall on the fovea, the deviated eye would remain deviated and not move.

Covering one eye forces the other to rotate in order to ____________.

186. $33\frac{1}{3}$ cm

187. If a fixation light is used as the target for phoria measurements at near, what method is best to disrupt fusion and dissociate the eyes?

335. 8

336. If a nonsquinting child with an ACA ratio of 4 and a hyperopia of 4 diopters looks at a target $33\frac{1}{3}$ cm away, he must accommodate a total of 7 diopters. Therefore, for a task at $33\frac{1}{3}$ cm this child develops 28 prism diopters of accommodative convergence.

A child with an ACA ratio of 4 and a hyperopia of 5 diopters must develop ____________ prism diopters of accommodative convergence when looking at a target $33\frac{1}{3}$ cm away.

484. V

485. The term **A** pattern esotrope is usually shortened to **A** esotrope. A **V** exotrope means that the patient is less exotropic in __________ gaze.

---

632. yes (but this impression has not been confirmed histologically)

633. There is a school of thought which teaches that most squints are caused by abnormal muscles or abnormal muscular attachments.

This theory holds that either abnormal (1) __________ or (2) __________ cause squints.

---

780. intermuscular membrane

781. If a muscle insertion is completely severed from the eyeball, it will not snap completely into the back of the orbit because it is held, to some extent, by the intermuscular membrane.

What prevents a muscle which is free of the eyeball from snapping into the back of the orbit?

38. get the target on the fovea

39. In esotropia, the eyes act as if they were improperly mounted in the sockets so that they are never aligned. When one eye is straight, the other eye is turned in; when the straight eye is covered, it then deviates inward by the amount that the other eye did when it was covered.

Does it matter which eye you allow to deviate in the measurement of the squint?

---

187. Maddox rod

188. What is the best means of dissociation if you wish to have accommodation stimulated by means of a reduced Snellen chart while testing the horizontal near phoria?

---

336. 32

337. If a child develops 28 prism diopters of accommodative convergence for a close task that requires 14 prism diopters of convergence, he must use 14 prism diopters of fusional divergence to keep the image on corresponding retinal points.

Fusional ____________ is used to overcome excessive accommodative convergence in people with straight eyes.

485. downward

486. A V esotrope may be straight in upward gaze, so the term **V** esotrope means that such an esotropia is present in __________ gaze.

633. (1) muscles } either
(2) attachments } order

634. In squint surgery, the various tendons attached to the eye muscles are cut, and the muscles themselves moved to a new position on the eyeball. In squint surgery, the (1) __________ are cut and the (2) __________ moved to new positions on the globe.

781. intermuscular membrane

782. If a muscle is completely severed from the eyeball, it will retract and probably reattach to the globe at an unpredictable distance behind its original insertion.

What becomes of an eye muscle if it is completely cut from its insertion on the globe?

39. no

40. As the eyes are alternately occluded, the occluded eye will instantly deviate an amount (equal to/greater than/less than) the deviation of the other eye when it was occluded.

188. vertical prism (about 6△)

189. Since accommodation stimulates convergence, an uncorrected hyperope would be expected to show (1) ____________ (what phoria), and plus lenses would be expected to (2) (reduce/increase) that phoria.

337. divergence

338. A child with a normal ACA ratio may have to overcome a great deal of accommodative convergence if he is a high hyperope.

High hyperopia even in the presence of a normal ACA ratio requires strong (1) ____________ divergence if (2) ____________ retinal points are to be stimulated.

486. downward

487. **V** esotropia means the tropia is greater on (1) ____________ gaze.

A esotropia means the tropia is greater on (2) ____________ gaze.

V exotropia means the tropia is greater on (3) ____________ gaze.

A exotropia means the tropia is greater on (4) ____________ gaze.

---

634. (1) ligaments (or tendons)
(2) muscles

635. How would squint surgery correct heavy check ligaments or abnormal adhesions?

---

782. It will probably reattach at an unpredictable distance behind the original insertion.

783. The tough, noncontractile portion of the muscle which inserts onto the eyeball is called the tendon. The ____________ of a muscle actually inserts onto the globe.

40. equal

41. If one eye turns in 40° while the other eye fixates a distant object straight ahead, the patient has an esotropia of ______°.

189. (1) esophoria
(2) reduce

190. An uncorrected myope would be expected to show (1) ______ (phoria) at near because less accommodation is used. The correct minus lenses would tend to (2) (increase/decrease) that phoria.

338. (1) fusional
(2) corresponding

339. If a child has a high ACA ratio or has a high hyperopia, he must have a strong fusional system to overcome the accommodative convergence and keep his eyes straight.

Accommodative convergence is present to an excessive degree in a patient with a high ACA ratio or high hyperopia. The excessive accommodative convergence must be overcome by a ______ if the patient is to keep his eyes straight.

487. (1) downward (3) upward
(2) upward (4) downward

488. The **A** and **V** patterns are present in about ¼ of all squints. Approximately ________ % of squints will have divergence or convergence differences of greater than 15△ between 25° upward and 25° downward gaze.

635. by cutting them (or similar wording)

636. There is a disease of the eye called **retinal detachment**. The treatment of this condition usually requires an operation on the back part of the eyeball. What is the usual treatment for retinal detachment?

783. tendon

784. If a muscle is severed from the globe at its insertion, the operation is called a tenotomy. A (1) ________ is an operation which severs the muscle from the globe at its (2) ________.

41. 40

42. If the esotrope is fixating a distant object, and the eyes are rapidly alternately occluded, the eye which is just uncovered will straighten to fixate while the eye which is just covered will deviate nasally. When an esotrope's straight eye is covered, it will turn (1) ____________, and the deviating eye will (2) ____________ when moving toward fixating an object straight ahead.

---

190. (1) exophoria
(2) decrease

191.

PART III
EXOTROPIA

(Advance to next frame.)

---

339. strong fusional system
(divergence fusional reserve)

340. The inherited tendency to squint plus an excessive amount of accommodative convergence usually team up to produce an accommodative esotropia.

An ____________ tendency is one component in producing an accommodative esotropia.

488. 25

489. A and V patterns of squints are detected by measuring the amount of squint present when the patient is gazing (1) ____________ and when
(direction and degrees)
gazing (2) ____________ .
(direction and degrees)

636. surgery

637. In order to reach the back half of the eye for surgery, a few of the eye muscles are usually detached from the globe early in the operation and then reattached at the close of the surgery.

In a retinal detachment operation, how is the back part of the eyeball reached?

784. (1) tenotomy
(2) insertion

785. Another method of weakening a muscle is to sever it through its meaty portion. Such a procedure is called a **myotomy**.

In a myotomy, the muscle is severed through its ____________ portion.

42. (1) in (or nasally)
(2) straighten (or turn out)

43. Ocular deviations are measured by comparing the actual position of an eye with the position that eye would have if it were properly sighting a specific target. The deviations are measured in relation to the actual position of an eye as compared to the ____________ position of that eye with respect to a specific target.

---

191. *(Advance to next frame.)*

192. In a patient with exotropia, we may see that sometimes the right eye turns out while the other eye fixates, and at other times the left eye turns out while the right looks at a target. The condition is called alternating exotropia.

In alternating exotropia (either eye/both eyes) may turn out at any one time.

---

340. inherited

341. If excessive hyperopia in an esotropic child (with a normal ACA ratio) is neutralized with the proper spectacles, his squint may disappear. Such a squint is called a totally accommodative esotropia.

If plus lenses straighten an esotrope's eyes, he is said to have a(n) ____________ accommodative esotropia.

489. (1) 25° up } either
(2) 25° down } order

490. Testing at positions of gaze greater than 25° from the straight ahead position is of little functional value, since patients usually turn their heads to see objects greater than 25° away from the straight ahead position. If an object is 40° from the straight ahead position, the patient will usually turn his ____________ to fixate the object.

637. by cutting some of the eye muscles at their attachment to the globe

638. One would expect many abnormal adhesions and imperfectly placed muscle insertions after retina surgery because of the extensive manipulations of the eye and muscles during the surgery.

What muscle abnormalities would you expect after retina surgery which might predispose to a squint?

785. meaty

786. Unfortunately, the eye muscles are not taut strings attached to a ball. Muscle tissue has an adaptability that strings and wire do not have. What characteristic might distinguish muscle tissue from string?

43. proper

44. Since some instruments measure squints in degrees, and others measure in prism diopters, a conversion from degrees to prism diopters is important. Approximately 2 prism diopters equal one degree. A 10° esotropia equals ____________ prism diopters esotropia.

192. either eye

193. In a case of exotropia, if the same eye always turns out, the case is defined as a monocular exotropia.

In monocular exotropia, the ____________ eye is always turned out.

341. totally

342. Most cases of accommodative esotropia are only partially straightened with glasses.

A hyperope whose esotropia lessens when he wears glasses is said to have a(n) ____________ accommodative esotropia.

490. head

491. Precise measurements of **A** and **V** patterns demand fixation 25° up and down. Extreme up and down gaze positions are helpful diagnostic positions, as the **A** and **V** patterns are accentuated in these extreme positions. In examining a patient for **A** and **V** patterns, the extreme positions are helpful for (1) ____________ purposes and the 25° up and down positions are important for (2) ____________ precisely the squint.

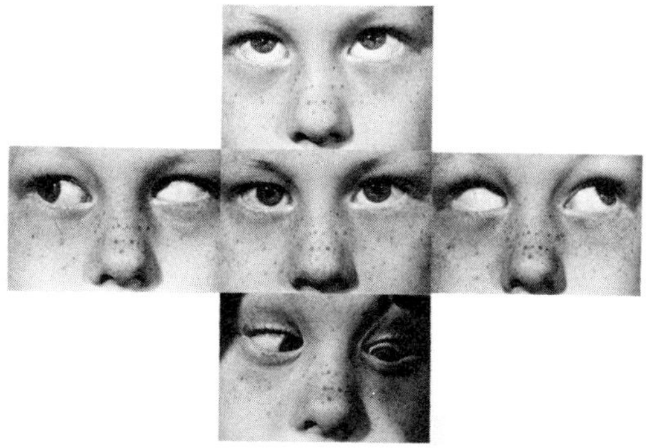

638. abnormal adhesions and inaccurately placed muscle insertions (or similar wording)

639. The development of a persistent squint is uncommon after retina surgery, even though retinal detachment surgery creates many abnormal muscle adhesions and incorrectly placed muscle insertions. Is persistent squint after retinal surgery common?

786. adaptability (ability to extend or contract)

787. A muscle's adaptability is due to the nerves and brain which control its movements and the inherent nature of muscle tissue.

List two factors responsible for a muscle's adaptability.

44. 20

45. 25△ (prism diopters) exotropia equals ________ ° exotropia.

193. same

194. An intermittent exotropia means that sometimes no squint is present and both eyes fixate on a target in a normal way. At other times, often when the patient is tired, one eye will turn out.

In a case of intermittent exotropia, the exotropia ________ constant.

342. partially

343. The term *partially accommodative esotropia* is meaningless as it tells only that the patient has some hyperopia. All patients, unless pathology is present, will have an esotropia reduced when plus lenses are placed in front of their eyes and some accommodation is reduced. A more appropriate classification is simply accommodative esotropia and esotropia with hyperopia. In front of a 3-diopter hyperopia, +3.00 lenses may not straighten his eyes, but the lenses will predictably ________ his esotropia.

491. (1) diagnostic } or equivalent
(2) measuring } wording

492. An **A** pattern esotropia is especially disturbing to the parents of a young child, for when the patient looks up at the parents the squint will be the ____________ .

639. no

640. It would appear that abnormal eye muscles can contribute to the cause of squint, but they cannot be considered the sole cause of squint.

Given moderately abnormal eye muscles or ligaments, list three other factors which might contribute to a squint.

787. (1) nerve and brain control } either
(2) inherent nature of muscle } order

788. The adaptability of muscle prevents a squint from being corrected by simply altering muscle pull by a mathematically predictable amount.

Mathematical analysis of the amount of muscle alteration needed to correct a squint is not that helpful because of the ____________ of muscle.

45. 12.5

46. This is a photo of 30△ exotropia (XT) or ______° XT.

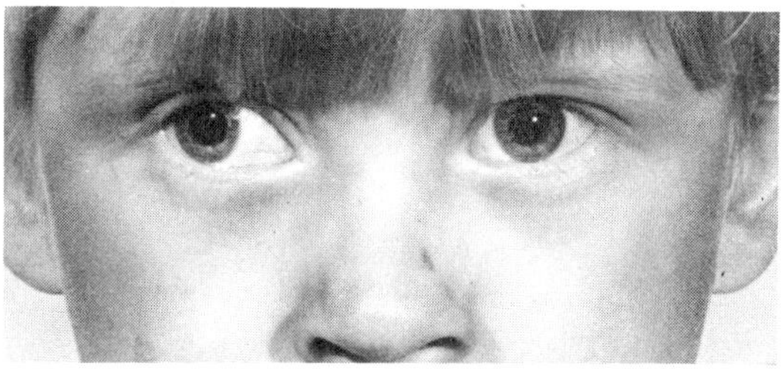

194. is not

195. Over one-half of the cases of exotropia are intermittent exotropia.

Of 100 exotropes, about how many will occasionally have straight eyes?

343. lessen or reduce

344. From the many investigations done on the incidence of different types of esotropia, it appears that about 50% of all esotropes can be made straight, for at least one distance, with glasses.

26% accom–Lyle
80% accom–Riggs
70% accom–Parks
30% accom–Kennedy
80% accom–Scobee
57% accom–Worth

About ______ % of all esotropes have a major accommodative element.

492. most pronounced (or worst)

493. If the child is a **V** exotrope, the exotropia will be the most pronounced when the child looks ________, hence disturbing to his parents.

640. abnormal ACA; faulty fusion; birth trauma; heredity; brain damage; refractive error; nerve damage; paresis of a vertical acting muscle; abnormal optomotor reflex; monocular vision (any three in any order)

641. Genetic studies have shown that a predisposition for overt squint is inherited. At present, we cannot be more specific.

The causative factor of squint is not known, but the predisposition for strabismus is________.

788. adaptability

789. About one-half of all cases of squint appear to have straight eyes when under general anesthesia before any surgery is done.

It is difficult to reduce squint surgery to simple mathematics, particularly in light of the fact that about ________ of the cases become straight under general anesthesia.

46. 15

47. One method of measuring a squint consists of having the patient look at an object directly in front of one eye, and then moving a flashlight along a calibrated arc until reflection of the light is seen in the center of the cornea of the deviating eye.

The patient has (1) ______________ ° (2) ______________ tropia.

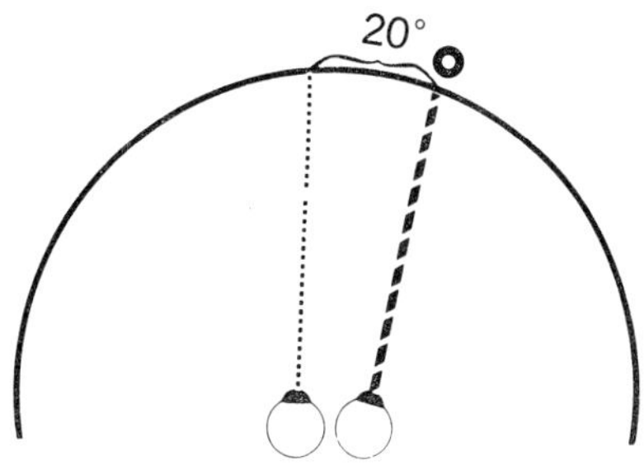

195. 50 (or over)

196. A case of intermittent exotropia may also be an alternating exotropia.

An exotropic patient may have a(n) (1) ______________ exotropia and a(n) (2) ______________ exotropia.

344. 50

345. Of all esotropes, about 10% are of the completely accommodative type.

27% Worth 77% Riggs 15% Scobee 6% Kennedy 7% Lyle	Various authors' estimation of totally accommodative esotropes

Of 100 children with esotropia, about ______________ will become straight at all times and at all distances with the proper glasses.

493. up

494. From the child's cosmetic viewpoint, upward gaze is most important, but from a functional point of view it is more important to have fusion in ____________ gaze where most of the work is accomplished.

641. inherited

642. It appears that if you inherit the squint factor, you may not necessarily squint, but you are prone to squint.

If you inherit the factor to squint, will you definitely squint?

789. one-half

790. Esotropia can be considered as an overaction of the medial recti. Recession of a medial rectus is often used to correct an esotropia. If the medial recti in an esotrope are attacked surgically, what procedure should be done?

47. (1) 20
(2) exo

48. The diagrammed patient has an (1) ____________ tropia of (2) ____________°.

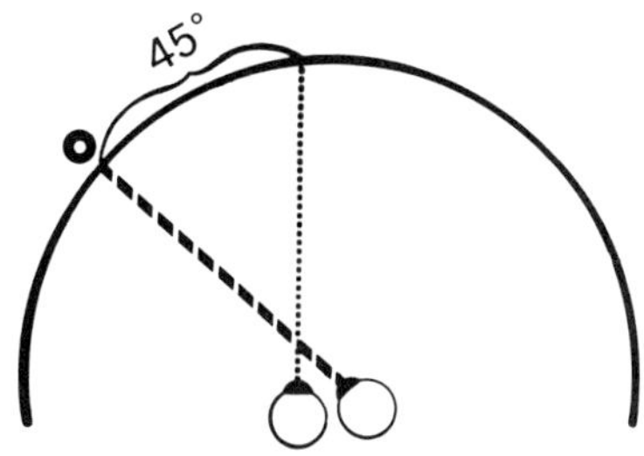

196. (1) alternating (or monocular) } either order
(2) intermittent

197. An exotropia is considered to be the comitant form if the deviating eye is misaligned by the same amount for any direction of gaze.

If one eye of an exotrope deviates 30° laterally from a target, irrespective of where the target is held, the exotropia is a ____________ form.

345. 10

346. Since about 10% of esotropes are totally accommodative, at least 90% of all esotropes will not be helped partially or completely by the proper glasses.

90% of all esotropes will not be helped by glasses because they are of the ____________ accommodative type.

494. downward

495. A V intermittent exotropic child who is 45° XT in upward gaze, but fuses in downward gaze, would be considered (1) __________ cosmetically, but (2) __________ functionally.

642. no

643. The presence of the squint factor plus the presence of another predisposing characteristic such as: (a) high hyperopia, (b) anisometropia, (c) poor fusion, (d) vertical acting muscle paresis, or (e) abnormal eye muscle would produce a squint.

Why don't all high hyperopes develop esotropia?

790. recession

791. It has been found that a constant amount of recession of the medial rectus (for example, 6 mm) will have different correcting effects on different sized esotropias.

Does recessing one medial rectus 4 mm have a constant effect on all sizes of esotropia?

48. (1) eso
(2) 45

49. The quantity of the squint can be estimated by noting the position of the corneal reflex (reflection of light on the cornea) when the patient fixates a light. Each mm the reflex is from the visual axis equals 15$^{\Delta}$. If the corneal reflex is in the center of one eye and 2 mm temporal to the center of the other eye (the eye is turned in), the patient will have approximately (1) ____________ (2) ____________ .
(amount) (type squint)

197. comitant

198. All forms of exotropia constitute about 20% of all the cases of squint.

In a group of 100 cases of squint, how many cases of exotropia would you probably find?

346. non

347. Since the accommodation through accommodative convergence plays some role in all esotropes, the exact status of refraction should be determined in all esotropes.

A ____________ should be part of the work-up in all esotropes.

495. (1) unsatisfactory
(2) satisfactory

496. An **A** esotropic child who is 45° ET in upward gaze, but fuses on downward gaze, may be cosmetically (1) ____________ , but functionally (2) ____________ .

---

643. Only those with the inherited squint factor or other predisposing factors will develop esotropia (or similar wording).

644.

PART IX
AMBLYOPIA

(Advance to next frame.)

---

791. no

792. Usually a 6 mm recession of the medial rectus will have a larger effect in a large esotropia than in a small ET.

If a 6 mm recession of a medial rectus has a 20 prism diopter effect in an ET of 25△, will it have a smaller, larger, or similar effect in an ET of 50△?

49. (1) 30△
(2) esotropia

50. The method of estimating a squint by means of 1 mm deviations of the corneal reflex equaling 15△ is known as the Hirshberg type of measurement. If the corneal reflex is 3 mm nasal to the center of one cornea (eye thus turned out), the patient has approximately (1) __________ (amount) (2) __________ (type squint) as estimated by the (3) __________ technique.

198. 20

199. In the case illustrated, the patient is looking straight ahead. Which eye is turned out?

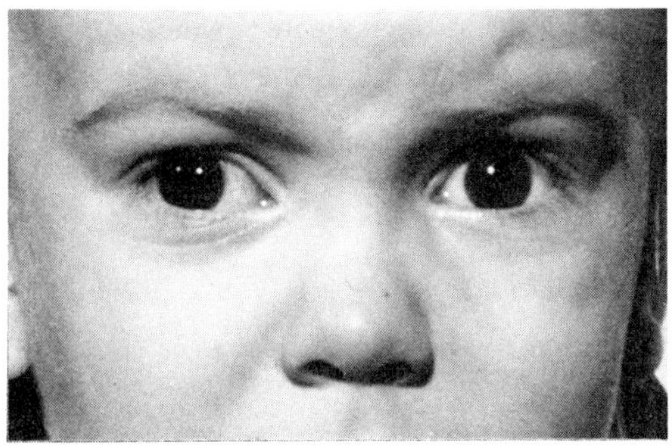

347. refraction

348. The total refractive error refers to the eye's optical state when no accommodation is used.

In measuring a patient's distance refractive error, all __________ should be eliminated.

496. (1) unsatisfactory
(2) satisfactory

497. **A** exotropia and **V** esotropia in children may have the reverse effects from the **V** exotropes and **A** esotropes; namely that, from the cosmetic viewpoint, the **A** exotropes and the **V** esotropes are satisfactory to their parents, but from a functional point of view they could not fuse in downward gaze and would be ____________.

---

644. *(Advance to next frame.)*

645. **Amblyopia** refers to poor vision in an eye (with refractive error corrected) which appears to have no organic disease.

How would the retina appear in a case of amblyopia?

---

792. larger

793. Voluntary muscles (such as the eye muscles) have certain properties. For example, a muscle put under stretch will contract more vigorously than a muscle which is not stretched.

As a voluntary muscle is stretched, it develops (larger/smaller) contractions.

50. (1) 45△
(2) exotropia
(3) Hirshberg

51. The corneal reflex is seen at the lateral limbus of one eye and in the center of the other (the corneal diameter is 12 mm). Utilizing the Hirshberg measurement the patient has approximately (1) __________ (2) __________.
(amount) (type squint)

199. OD (right)

200. In the illustration, the patient with exotropia is looking at an object straight ahead and close to him. Which eye is not able to converge enough?

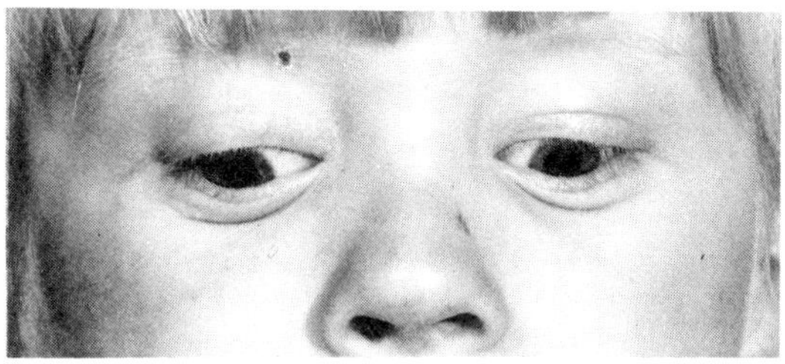

348. accommodation

349. In a child, the best way to eliminate accommodation is to paralyze the ciliary body.

A drug which paralyzes the ciliary body eliminates __________.

497. unsatisfactory

498. These illustrations show a(n) (1) __________ pattern (2) __________ .

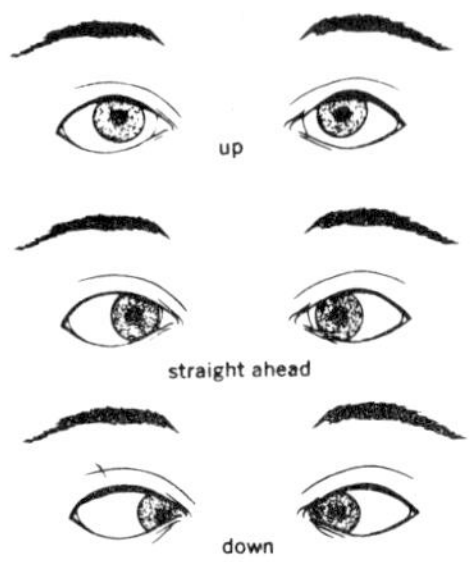

645. normal

646. In general, only one eye is amblyopic; the other eye retains normal vision.

Is it common to encounter amblyopia in both eyes?

793. larger

794. It is also known that if a voluntary muscle is stretched, it will develop more tension when stimulated than a muscle which is not stretched.

How does the stretch of a muscle affect the tension which develops in that muscle when it is stimulated?

51. (1) 90△ (or 45°)
(2) esotropia

52. When the corneal reflex is about halfway nasally from the center of the cornea to the limbus (3 mm from the center), and the reflex is in the center of the other cornea, the patient has (1) ________ (amount) (2) ________ (type squint) as measured by the (3) ________ method.

---

200. OD (right)

201. A patient with a constant amount of exotropia has one eye which turns out when looking at a distant object. When looking at a near object, both eyes converge, but one eye doesn't converge enough; therefore, it still appears turned out compared to the other eye. A patient with exotropia (can/cannot) converge the turned eye to some extent when changing fixation from a distant object to a near object.

---

349. accommodation

350. The Greek term **cyclo** means "circle" or "wheel" and has come to refer to the ciliary body because of its circular arrangement. The Greek term **plegia** means "paralysis."

A cycloplegic drug (1) ________ the (2) ________ body.

498. (1) V
(2) esotrope

499. These illustrations show a(n) (1) __________ pattern (2) __________ . (The patient is orthophoric on downward gaze.)

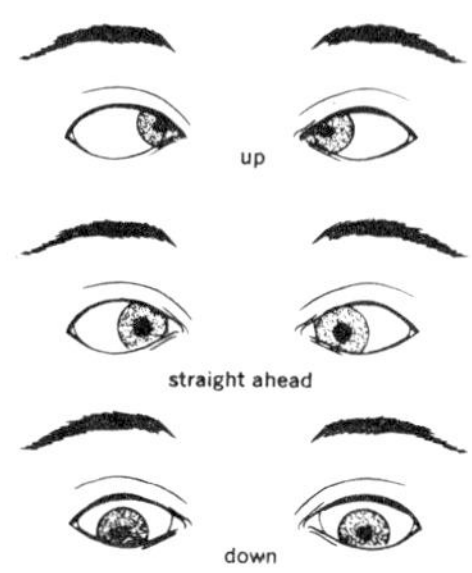

646. no

647. It is generally accepted that amblyopia is present if the best corrected vision in one eye is at least 2 lines poorer on the Snellen chart than the other eye and no organic pathology is seen.

From the following recorded visual acuity, which eye has the amblyopia (if no organic disease is present)?

OD 20/20
OS 20/40

794. The greater the stretch, the greater the tension (or similar wording).

795. The relationship between stretch and tension in a muscle is shown in the graph. When a muscle is stretched, the tension developed during stimulation increases proportionally. As the stretch is increased, the tension increases at an even greater rate until the muscle is overstretched and develops less tension. The graph of the tension-stretch relationship shows X representing the stretch and Y representing __________ .

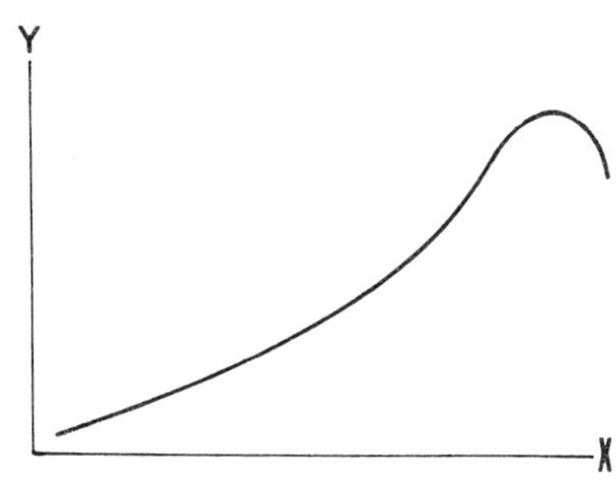

52. (1) 45△
(2) exotropia
(3) Hirshberg

53. This photo shows an (1) ____________ (type squint) measuring approximately (2) ____________ △ by the Hirshberg method.

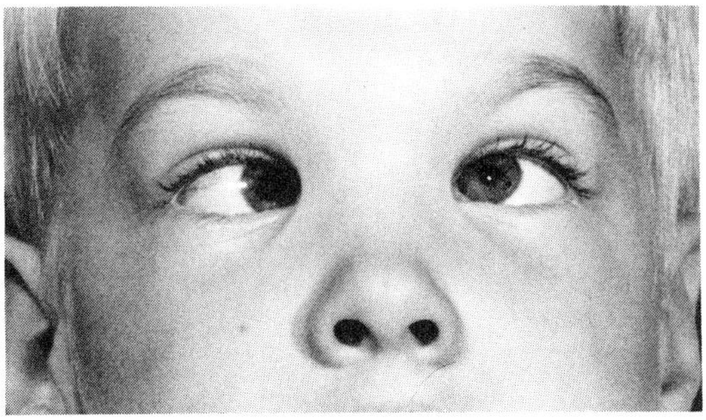

201. can

202. If both eyes appear to look at a distant object properly, but one eye turns out when the patient attempts to converge his eyes to a close object, the patient is said to be exotropic at near. Patients who are exotropic only at near have (1) ____________ eyes with distant fixation but are (2) ____________ with near fixation.

350. (1) paralyzes
(2) ciliary

351. Drugs like atropine, homatropine, and cyclopentolate are cycloplegic drugs. ____________ is one drug used for a cycloplegic refraction.

499. (1) **A**
(2) esotrope

500. These illustrations show a(n) (1) ______ pattern (2) ______.

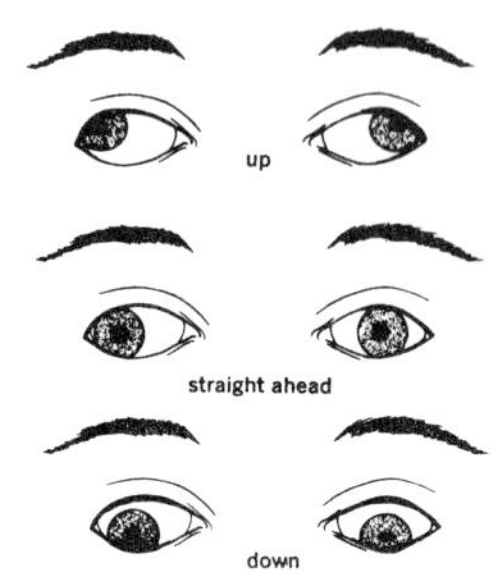

647. OS

648. The incidence of amblyopia in the general population is similar to that of squint, that is about ______ %.

(Refer to Table 1 preceding index.)

795. tension (produced by the muscle)

796. When a muscle is recessed, it is stretched less. Therefore, when it is stimulated, its amplitude of contraction is less.

When an eye muscle is ______, a given amount of stimulation produces less contraction than in an unoperated muscle.

53. (1) esotrope
(2) 75△ (± 15△)

54. This photo shows an (1) ____________ which (type squint) measures approximately (2) ____________ (amount) by the (3) ____________ method.

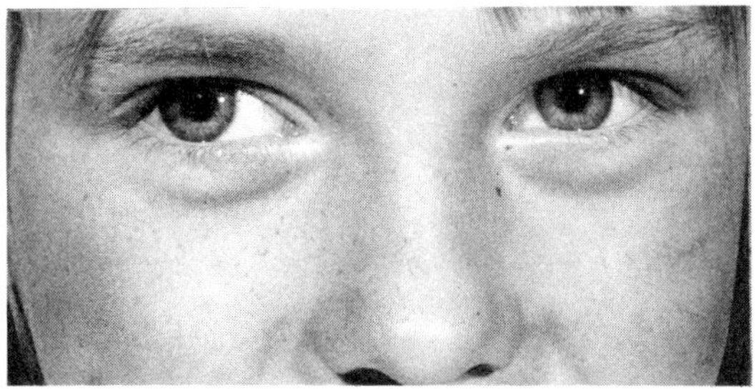

202. (1) straight
(2) exotropic (or divergent)

203. A patient who has straight eyes while fixating a distant object, but is exotropic when looking at objects nearby, has an inability to converge adequately called convergence insufficiency.

A patient who is ortho at distance but 20△ XT′ probably has ____________ .

351. either: atropine
homatropine
cyclopentolate

352. In an esotropic child a cycloplegic examination is important in covering all the hyperopia present. The greatest plus that will give reasonably clear distance vision can be prescribed and the glasses' effect on the esotropia noted.

In determining the maximum hyperopic correction in a child a(n) ____________ refraction should be performed.

500. (1) V
(2) exotrope

501. These illustrations show a(n) (1)____________ pattern (2) ____________.

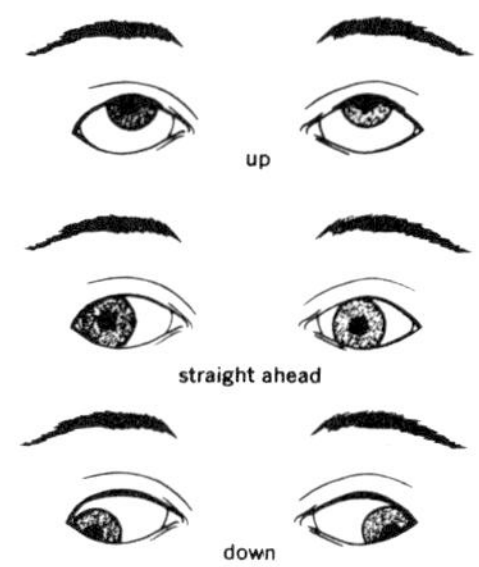

648. 2

649. Amblyopia is often linked with strabismus, and it is estimated that about ____________ % of strabismus cases have amblyopia.

(Refer to Table 1.)

796. recessed

797. When one eye muscle is recessed, the muscles pulling the opposite way have less opposition and are also stretched less.

If the medial rectus is recessed, does the opposing lateral rectus become (more/less) stretched?

54. (1) exotropia
(2) $45^{\triangle}$ ($\pm$ $15^{\triangle}$), or $25°$ ($\pm$ $8°$)
(3) Hirshberg

55. The Hirshberg measurement of squints is done by ___________.
(how calculated)

203. convergence insufficiency

204. Convergence insufficiency implies that the patient cannot ___________ adequately to maintain fusion at near.

352. cycloplegic

353. However, before getting too enthusiastic in finding a hyperopic condition in a child, it should be realized that the average refractive error for a normal group of 3-year-olds is about 3 diopters of hyperopia.

The average refractive error for 3-year-olds is ___________.
(amount and type)

501. (1) **A**
(2) exotrope

502. The cause of **V** and **A** patterns of squints is not known, but empirical surgical treatments have been devised. The cause of **A** and **V** patterns is ____________.

649. 50

650. Anisometropia refers to the asymmetry of the refractive status of the two eyes.

What term would best describe a condition in which one eye was myopic and the other eye hyperopic?

797. less

798. Anatomic studies show a wide variation between the thickness of specific muscles in various individuals.

Would the medial rectus be the same size in all individuals?

55. noting the position of the corneal reflex and allowing 15△ for each mm deviation from the center of the cornea (or equivalent wording)

56. The amplitude of an exotropia can be measured if we can measure the angle between the visual axes. If the visual axes form an angle of 45° behind the head, then the patient has an exotropia of ____________°.

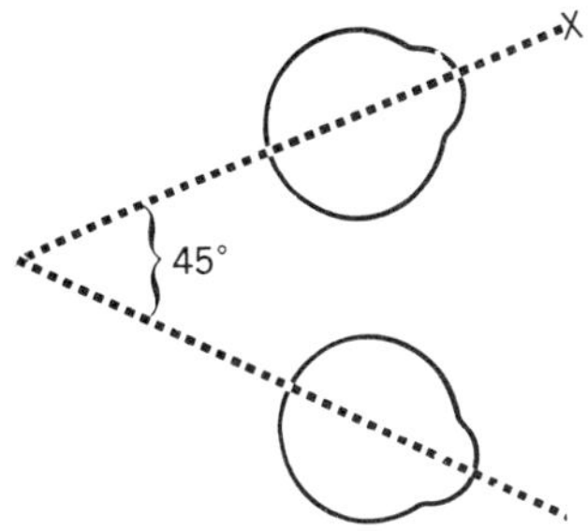

204. converge

205. Convergence insufficiency implies that the patient converges less with accommodation than the normal. A patient with convergence insufficiency will be expected to have a (high/low) ACA ratio.

353. 3.00 D of hyperopia

354. Although applying a hyperopic correction for 3 diopters or less in an esotrope may alter his squint, your chances of curing a squint with glasses are better in higher hyperopes.

Most accommodative esotropes have a hyperopia of greater than ____________.

502. not known

503. An important objective in the treatment of **A** and **V** pattern squints is to avoid making the patient worse. You might hesitate before instituting any surgical treatment in (1) ____________ exotropes or (2) ____________ esotropes who could fuse on downward gaze.

650. anisometropia

651. Although slight differences in refraction between the two eyes are common, anisometropia is usually considered significant if a difference of 2.0 diopters or more exists.

If a patient had emmetropia in OD, what refraction would he have to have in OS to be considered to have significant anisometropia?

798. no

799. Although muscle size varies in different individuals, the medial rectus is generally longer, thicker and more powerful than the lateral rectus in the same individual.

Of the horizontal rectus muscles, which is the largest?

56. 45

57. Methods are available to allow each eye to have a separate fixation target.

OS sees (1) ______________ .
(sketch)

OD sees (2) ______________ .
(sketch)

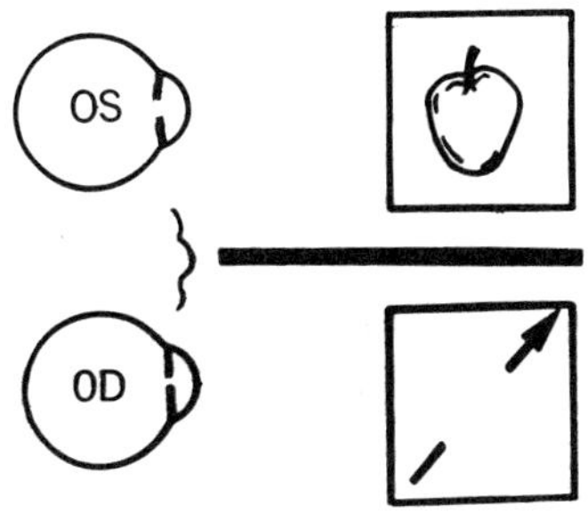

205. low

206. A patient with convergence insufficiency has a low ACA ratio; however, he will have a (smaller/greater) XT′ at near if he can be made to accommodate more at near.

354. 3 diopters

355. There are a number of other characteristics seen in both accommodative and nonaccommodative esotropes which often help in determining diagnosis.

Some children squint all the time and are called constant, others periodically, usually when fatigued.

Squints may be classified as either intermittent or ______________ .

503. (1) **V**
(2) **A**

504. The cosmetic features of **A** and **V** pattern squints should be considered secondary to the functional requirements, for as the child grows taller the cosmetic effect of upward gaze of the child will ____________ .

---

651. at least 2.0 diopters of myopia or hyperopia or astigmatism } any one

652. The incidence of anisometropia of 2.0 diopters or more is about ____________ % in the general population.

(Refer to Table 1.)

---

799. medial rectus

800. We are now in a position to understand why a recession of the medial rectus has a greater effect than an equal amount of resection of the lateral rectus in the case of ET.

In the treatment of ET, does a recession of the medial rectus or a resection of the lateral rectus have a greater effect?

57. 1.  2. 

58. If fixation objects are shown each eye independently, as occlusion is alternated the eyes will not deviate if the objects are placed at the angle of squint along the visual axis of each eye.

Alternate occlusion, with objects on visual axes, results in (some/no) movement of the eyes.

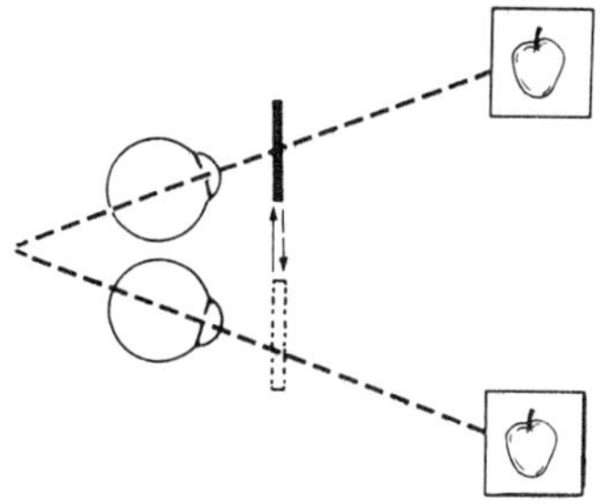

---

206. smaller

207. Since a patient with convergence insufficiency has a low ACA ratio, we wish him to accommodate as much as possible. Any hyperopia would be better (corrected/uncorrected) to stimulate all accommodation possible at near.

---

355. constant

356. The intermittent squint is straight periodically. When his eyes are straight, an observed target falls on corresponding points of both retinas, and he is said to have fusion.

An intermittent esotrope has fusion when his eyes are ______________.

504. be less noticeable (or equivalent words)

505. In 1897, Duane reported a patient with bilateral superior oblique paresis who was orthophoric on upward gaze, but markedly esotropic on downward gaze. This was a (1) __________ pattern (2) __________ caused by bilateral paresis of the (3) __________ .

---

652. 2

653. Just as in squint, about __________ % of the patients with significant anisometropia have amblyopia.

(Refer to Table 1.)

---

800. recession of the medial rectus

801. A recession of the medial rectus decreases the stretch on both the bigger medial rectus and the less powerful lateral rectus. Thus the operation decreases the contractile power of the medial rectus more than the lateral rectus.

If the medial rectus can develop a force of 1000 gm, and the lateral rectus a force of 800 gm, and each is weakened by 10%, how much force does each muscle lose?

58. no

59. The amblyoscope is one of a class of instruments called haploscopes, stereoscopes, or diploscopes. These instruments allow placement of a target along the visual axis of each eye. The effect of occlusion is made by illuminating each target independently.

The amblyoscope allows alternate fixation of targets along the ____________ of each eye at any angle of squint.

207. uncorrected

208. The term asthenopia is used to cover a broad category of symptoms such as a general sense of discomfort, mild headaches, and a mild aching of the eyes. Phorias may occasionally cause such symptoms. If large phorias are found in a patient with asthenopic symptoms you (would, would not) treat such phorias.

356. straight

357. If an esotrope has fusion, his chances of having straight eyes after treatment are much higher than if he had never demonstrated fusion.

The presence of ____________ improves the prognosis of the treatment of the esotrope.

505. (1) V
(2) esotrope
(3) superior oblique

506. When the superior obliques are paretic, the inferior obliques seem to be capable of overacting, thus turning the eyes out excessively in upward gaze. Thus, in **V** esotropes, we should look for overaction of the (1) ____________ muscles or underaction of the (2) ____________ muscles.

653. 50

654. It has also been noted that if a patient has a squint and anisometropia, his chances for having amblyopia are greater.

(See Table 1.)

The simultaneous occurrence of (1) ____________ and (2) ____________ increases the incidence of amblyopia.

801. MR–100 gm
LR – 80 gm

802. A recession weakens the pull of each horizontal rectus, but the medial rectus loses more than the lateral rectus.

In a recession operation of the medial rectus, which muscle loses more power, the medial or lateral rectus?

59. visual axis

60. The fixation objects can be varied easily with an amblyoscope until the point is reached where the eyes do not move when they are alternately occluded. The angle the visual axes make with each other can then be read directly from the amblyoscope. This angle is the ___________ of the squint.

208. would

209. Convergence insufficiency may cause asthenopic symptoms when near work is attempted. Additional fusional convergence can be developed with appropriate exercises.

To treat convergence insufficiency, ___________ should be developed with appropriate exercises.

357. fusion

358. Roughly 50% of all esotropes will sometimes cross the right eye, using the left eye to fixate, and at other times cross the left eye, directing the right eye to an object of interest.

___________ % of esotropes are considered alternators.

506. (1) inferior oblique
(2) superior oblique

507. The same oblique muscles are incriminated in **V** esotropia as in **V** exotropia. Just as excessive turning in of the eyes on downward gaze in **V** esotropia may be caused by overaction of the inferior obliques or underaction of the superior obliques, so in **V** exotropia the relative inturning of the eye in downward gaze may be caused by overaction of the (1) ____________ or underaction of the (2) ____________ .

---

654. (1) anisometropia } either
(2) squint } order

655. The two basic categories of amblyopia are the amblyopes associated with squint and the amblyopes associated with anisometropia. Amblyopia is commonly associated with either (1) ____________ or (2) ____________ .

---

802. medial rectus

803. In a resection of the lateral rectus, increased stretch is placed on both the medial rectus and the lateral rectus.

Does a resection increase or decrease the stretch of the horizontal recti?

60. angle (or amount)

61. In essence, the amblyoscope has targets which can be alternately illuminated (same effect as alternately occluding the eyes). The targets are moved with constant alternate flashing until ____________ movement of the eyes is seen with each alternate illumination.

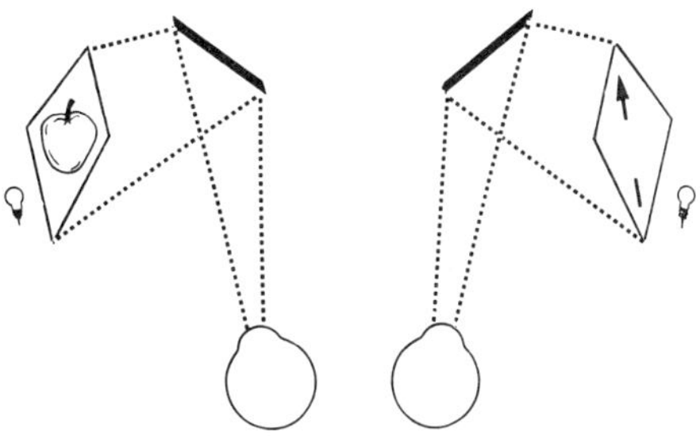

209. additional fusional convergence (fusional convergence)

210. Fusional convergence can be developed by teaching the patient to converge on objects progressively closer to his eyes while maintaining binocular vision. To develop additional fusional convergence, the patient must use ____________ eye(s) during any training periods.

358. 50

359. The tendency of some esotropes to alternate is manifested by the esotrope looking at any fixation object on his left with his right eye and any object on his right with his left eye. This is known as cross fixating.

The diagram illustrates an esotrope who is ____________ .

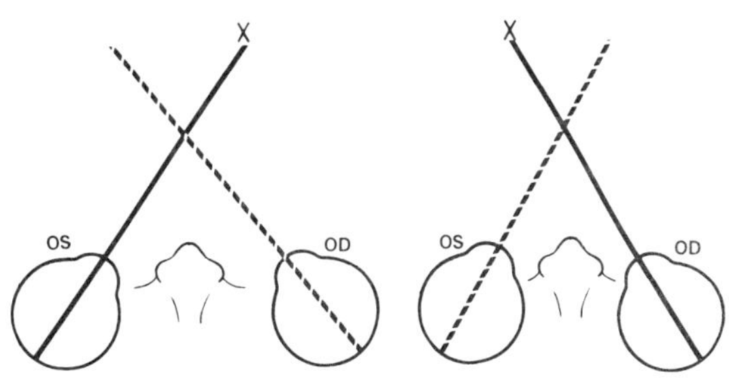

507. (1) inferior obliques
(2) superior obliques

508. Overaction of the inferior obliques can be demonstrated by directing the patient's gaze to either side and noting the upward deviation of the adducting eye.

The photos demonstrate overaction of both ____________.

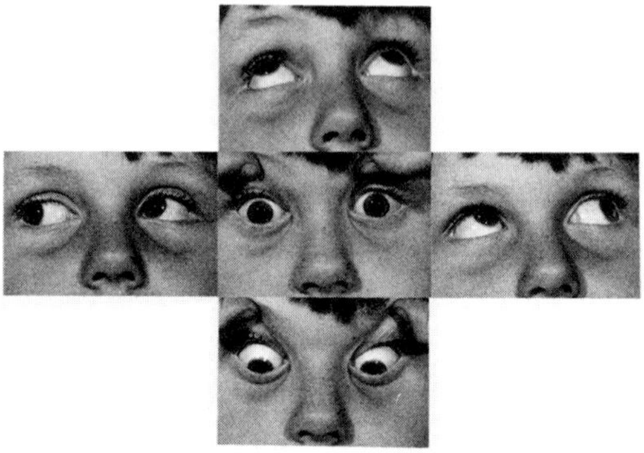

655. (1) squint
(2) anisometropia } either order

656. Normally we do not use all of both retinas simultaneously. This tendency to use one area of one retina, then a corresponding area of the other, is called retinal rivalry.

The alternate use of portions of each retina is called ____________.

803. increase

804. In a lateral rectus resection, although the eye is repositioned temporally, the medial rectus achieves greater power when it contracts.

What is the effect on the contraction of the medial rectus when the lateral rectus is resected?

61. no

62. If the amblyoscope has to be set so that the tubes diverge 10° from parallel before deviations of the eye cease when alternately occluded, the patient has (1) ________ ° (2) ________ tropia.

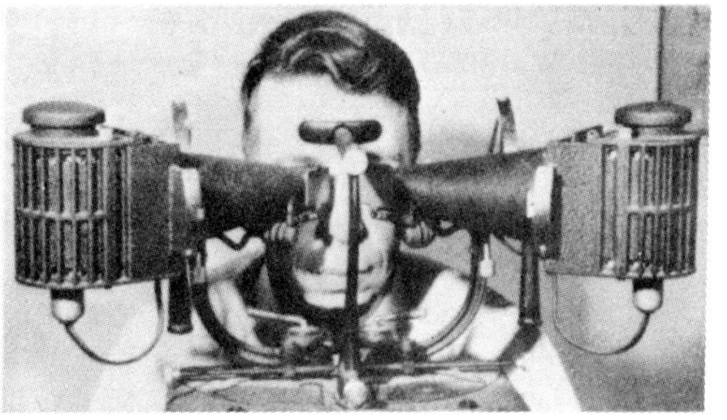

210. both

211. The patient is taught to constantly check whether he is using both eyes in any fusional convergence training. To check on the use of both eyes, the patient must have some clue. For example, if the patient tries to bring the tip of a pencil closer and closer to his nose, a different color pencil should be held farther away. The image of the pencil held farther away will fall on noncorresponding retinal points, and the patient will see ________ images of the distant pencil.

359. cross fixating

360. An esotrope who fixates objects on his right with his left eye and fixates objects on his left with his right eye is known as a ________ fixator.

508. inferior obliques

509. The results of strengthening procedures of the superior oblique muscle are hard to predict, so weakening surgery on the inferior oblique is preferred in (1) ____________ esotropia and (2) ____________ exotropia to convert the incomitant squint (the **V** pattern) to a comitant squint in the esotrope and to straighten the exotrope.

656. retinal rivalry

657. The pattern (is/is not) seen as a grid due to retinal rivalry.

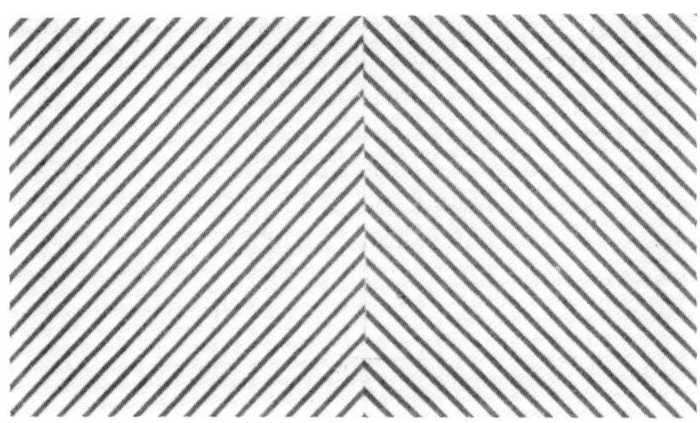

Retinal rivalry is demonstrated by having different patterns presented to each eye. If you can cross your eyes, notice how you will see patches of lines going in one direction or the other but never overlapping lines.

804. Contraction power is increased.

805. The recession operation in ET repositions the eye outward and weakens the contraction of the medial rectus more than the lateral rectus. The resection operation in ET repositions the eye outward but strengthens the contraction of the medial rectus more than the lateral rectus.

Is the recession of the medial rectus or the resection of the lateral rectus more effective in ET?

62. (1) 10
(2) exo

63. The (1) ____________ is an instrument which measures angles of squint by alternately illuminating movable targets until no eye movement is seen.

The (2) ____________ of squint can be read directly from the instrument's scale.

211. two

212. The patient attempts to bring one pencil closer to his nose while seeing two images of the pencil held farther away. He sees only one image of the nearer pencil if he is aligning his foveas because the images of the near pencil strike ____________ areas on the retina.

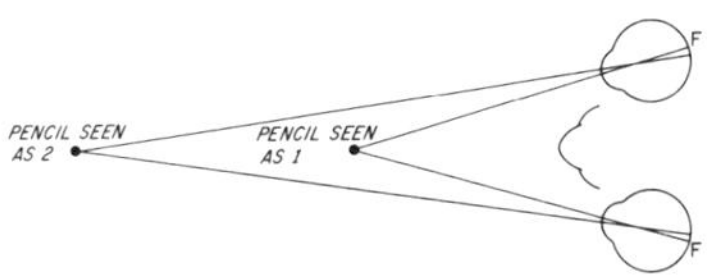

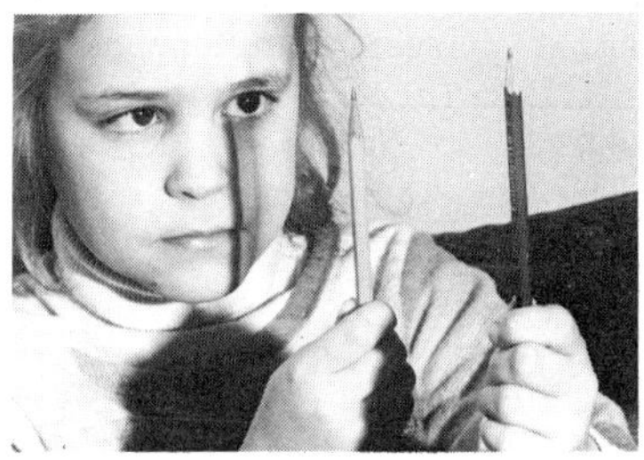

360. cross

361. Generally speaking, alternating esotropes have equally good vision in both eyes, since they use either eye indiscriminately.

Usually alternating esotropes have ____________ vision in both eyes.

509. (1) **V**
(2) **V**

510. Overaction of the inferior obliques or underaction of the superior obliques has been incriminated in **V** esotropes or **V** exotropes. The oblique muscles have been incriminated also in **A** esotropes and **A** exotropes, where the superior obliques can be demonstrated frequently to be overacting or the inferior obliques to be ____________ occasionally.

657. is not

658. The preceding frame demonstrated the normal inability to appreciate two dissimilar retinal images simultaneously and is called ____________.

805. recession of medial rectus

806. The diagram shows a portion of a slide rule.

Notice how the lower end of the scale is wide, whereas lots of squeezing together occurs at the ____________ end of the scale.

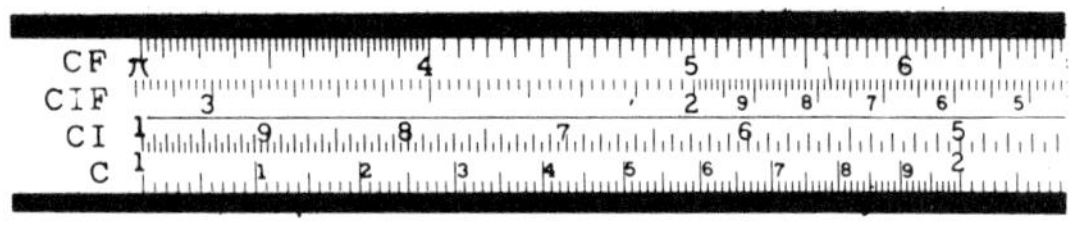

63. (1) amblyoscope
(2) angle (or amount)

64. We can also measure squints by using prisms.

Whereas a plane sheet of glass allows a ray of light to pass through it in a straight fashion (*A*), a prism bends a ray of light (*B*).

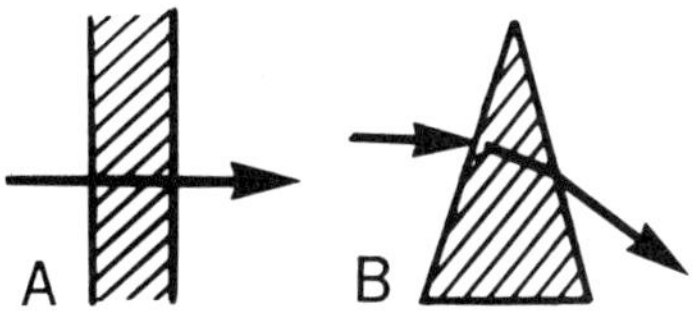

Light rays are bent by a ____________ .

212. corresponding (foveal)

213. The two-pencil fusional convergence exercise is easy to teach most patients. The patient is instructed to bring the pencil progressively closer to him and to try to still see the point singly while seeing two of the pencils held farther away. The single point may be blurred because the limit of accommodation, and hence accommodative convergence, has been exceeded and only fusional convergence is being used. Practice in the above would be expected to increase the patient's ____________ .

361. equal (equally good)

362. Esotropes are classified as alternating esotropes or monocular esotropes. Alternating esotropes cross either eye, but monocular esotropes cross the ____________ eye all the time.

510. underacting

511. Overaction of the superior obliques can be demonstrated by directing the patient to gaze to either side and noting a downward deviation of the adducting eye.

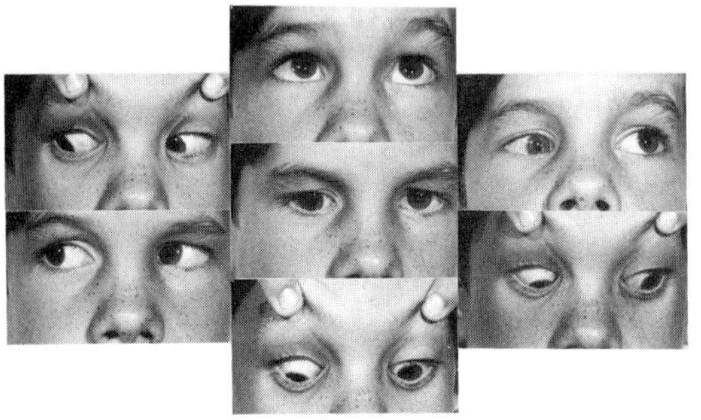

The photos demonstrate overaction of the ___________.

658. retinal rivalry

659. Retinal rivalry is a form of physiologic suppression. If there is a condition where one retinal image is continuously blurred, the rivalry will be a one-sided contest and the blurred image may be ___________.

806. upper

807. On the slide rule, a 1 mm space between eight and ten accounts for a big change of value, whereas the same distance between one and two accounts for a little change in value.

On the slide rule, does a 2 mm move represent a greater change at the lower or upper end of the scale?

64. prism

65. A prism always bends light rays in the direction of its base.

In figure *A*, light is bent toward the ______________, and in figure *B*, light is bent toward the (2) ______________ .

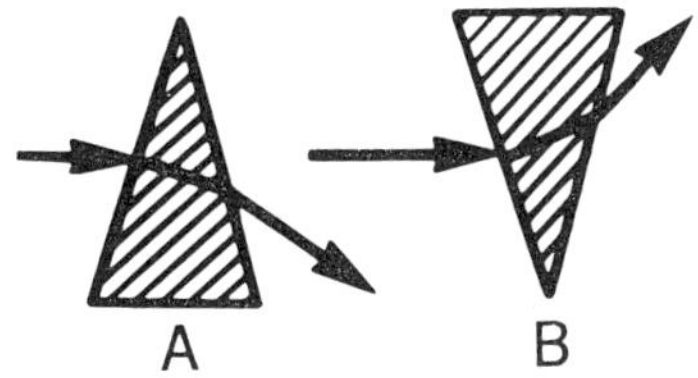

213. fusional convergence (reserve)

214. (*Turn to the back of the book and remove Panel 1.*) Another technique for teaching the patient to converge maximally while using both eyes is to look at a straight line held close to the nose as in the photo.

Hold Panel 1 in the same manner. Look at figure 5 on the line. You see the two lines form a letter ______________. (Be sure both eyes are open.)

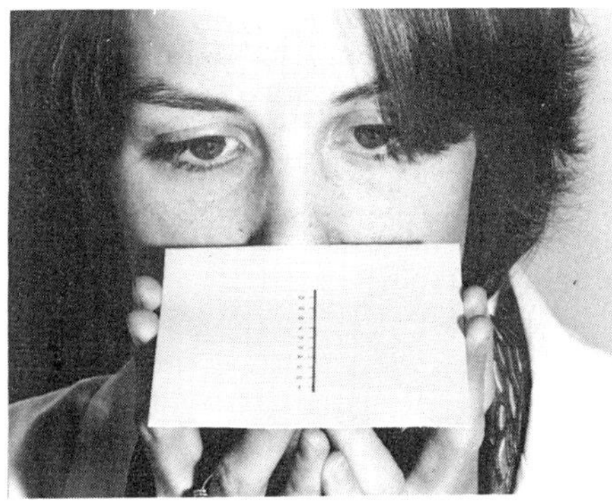

362. same

363. Although the results of different investigations of squints vary, it appears that the chances for permanently straight eyes are similar for alternating esotropes and monocular esotropes.

Prognosis is ______________ for alternating esotropes and monocular esotropes.

511. superior obliques

512. An easy way to remember which muscle is overacting is to recall that the inferior obliques overact in **V** patterns (the **V** points inferiorly), and that the superior obliques overact in **A** patterns (the **A** points superiorly).

In **V** patterns frequently the (1) ____________ overact.

In **A** patterns frequently the (2) ____________ overact.

---

659. suppressed

660. In squint, the deviating eye may suppress vision to avoid diplopia. In anisometropia, the eye with the greater refractive error may suppress vision to avoid a confusing blur.

The act of ____________ is common in the deviating eye in squint and in the more ametropic eye in anisometropia.

---

807. upper

808. In a logarithmic relationship such as on a slide rule, an effect is not constant over the entire scale but takes on greater importance at the upper end of the scale.

The slide rule is an example of a ____________ relationship.

65. (1) base
(2) base

66. In the illustration, the prism is placed with its base facing the side of the head. This is known as placing a prism base-out.

If a prism is placed before the eye with its base out, is the base toward the temple or the nose?

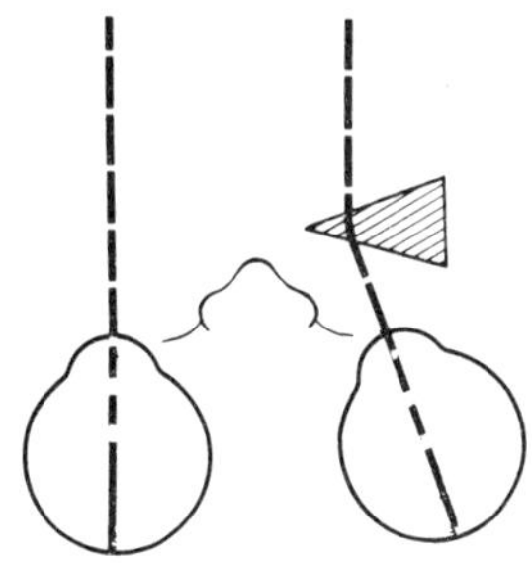

214. *X*

215. To converge maximally, the patient is first asked to look close to point 1 on the line. If he is using both eyes, he should see an inverted v. Try this yourself with Panel 1. You will see the lines as depicted, forming a(n) ____________ .

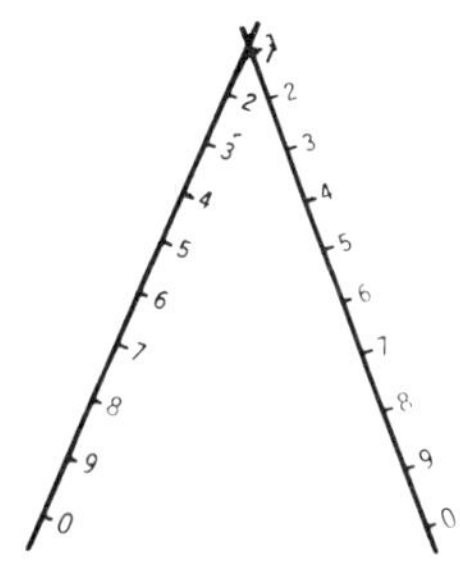

363. similar

364. Some esotropes squint the same amount all the time and are called fixed; others have different amounts of esotropia on different occasions.

Esotropia may be classified as being variable or ____________ .

512. (1) inferior obliques
(2) superior obliques

513. The actual cause of **A** and **V** patterns is not known, and the observation that obliques frequently overact in **A** and **V** patterns of squints does not mean that this is the cause of these patterns, for there are many **A** and **V** patterns in which no overaction or underaction of the obliques can be demonstrated. What is the cause of the **A** and **V** patterns of squint?

---

660. suppression

661. Some investigators feel that prolonged suppression of vision may eventually lead to amblyopia.

Amblyopia may be caused by ____________ .

---

808. logarithmic

809. The relationship of muscle stretch and tension development as illustrated in the graph is a logarithmic relationship.

Notice how gradual the slope of the curve is at *A*, and how ____________ it is near the peak *B*.

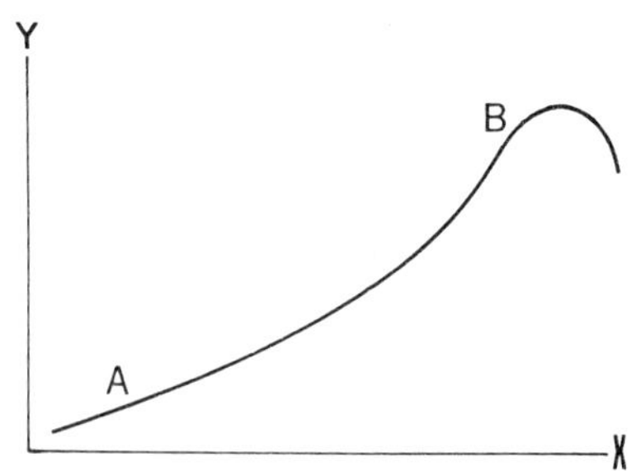

66. temple

67. In the illustration, the prism is placed in front of the eye with its base toward the nose. This is known as base-in.

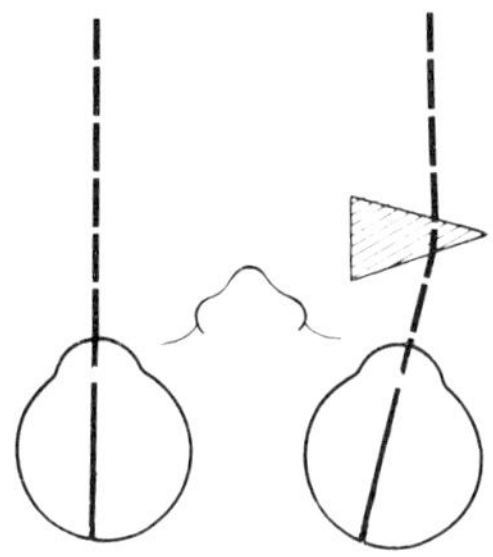

If a prism is placed before the eye with its base in, is the base facing the temple or the nose?

215. inverted v (or equivalent)

216. Using Panel 1 held close to you as before, look at point 5. You should see a figure, as depicted, forming a(n) ____________ .

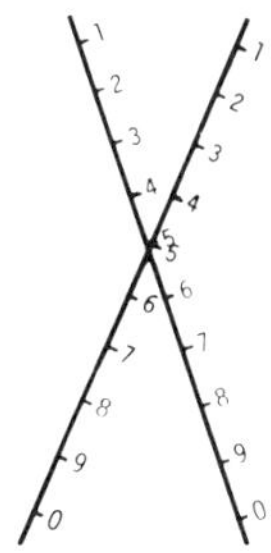

364. fixed

365. It appears that surgery done on a variable esotrope has a greater correcting effect than the same amount of surgery done on a fixed esotrope.

The same operation done on a variable esotrope has a ____________ effect than on a fixed esotrope.

513. The cause is not known.

514. Since a mild physiologic **V** pattern frequently exists, downward gaze seems to involve some stimulation to the medial recti. A **V** esotrope could be imagined to have overaction of the ___________ muscles (as well as overaction of the inferior obliques) in downward gaze.

661. prolonged suppression

662. Any disturbance of vision in about the first eight years of life may cause amblyopia. If the visual disturbance is asymmetric, the child is particularly prone to develop amblyopia. Congenital glaucoma is commonly unilateral as are congenital cataracts. Successful technical treatment of the unilateral congenital glaucoma and unilateral cataracts may result in an optically and an anatomically good cure, but that eye may not see well due to ___________.

809. steep

810. A muscle can develop greater tension either by being stretched or by receiving stronger stimulation from its nerve supply.

A muscle can develop a greater amplitude of contraction by being (1) ___________ at the time of contraction or by having stronger (2) ___________.

67. nose

68. Consider the properties of prisms.

Light is deflected toward the base of a prism. Object *A* in the diagram will appear to be located at position *B*. The object appears displaced toward the ____________ of the prism.

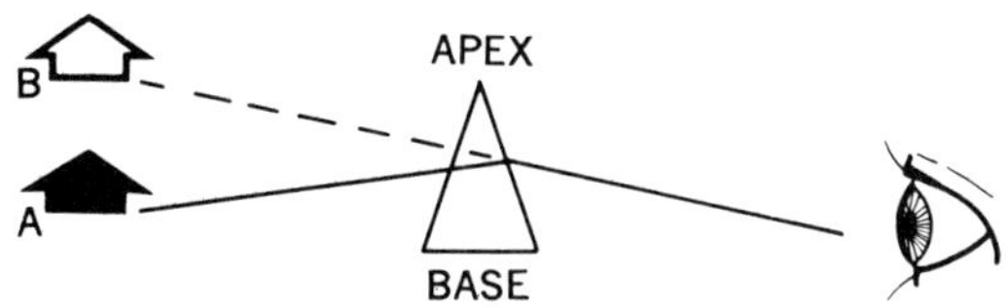

216. X

217. Look at 0 or 9. You see the lines forming a ____________, as depicted.

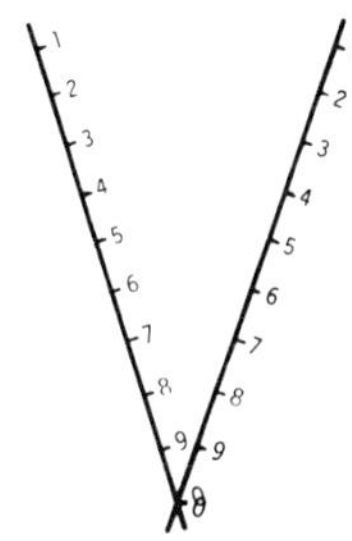

365. greater

366. Esotropes are considered concomitant if the amount of squint is the same no matter which direction they look.

A concomitant esotrope has the ____________ angle of squint regardless of the direction in which he turns his eyes.

514. medial rectus

515. A system for weakening the adducting power of the medial recti in the lower field of gaze consists of moving the muscle insertion down (usually 5 mm). To weaken the adducting power of the medial recti in downward gaze, move the insertion of the (1) __________ (2) __________ .
(muscle) (what direction)

662. amblyopia

663. Vision in the amblyopic eye can usually be restored if treatment is undertaken early. How does the duration of amblyopia affect the prognosis of the restoration of vision?

810. (1) stretched
(2) stimulation

811. If a muscle is near the upper end of its tension potential, small changes in stretch or nerve stimulation have proportionally greater effect on the tension than at low levels of tension.

If one medial rectus is contracted maximally, and a second medial rectus is contracted a little, in which will a 5 mm recession have a greater effect?

68. apex

69. When a horizontal line is observed through a prism, as diagrammed, the image of the line is displaced toward the ____________ of the prism.

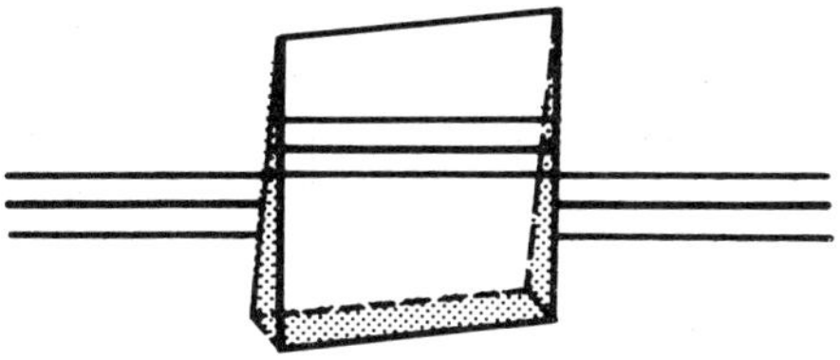

217. V

218. We have said that more than half of all exotropes are intermittent. When they are not squinting, both visual axes point to the same target, and the brain is able to integrate the information from both retinas in a normal fashion.

When an intermittent exotrope is straight, his brain is able to ____________ the information from both retinas in a normal fashion.

366. same

367. A noncomitant esotrope alters his angle of squint in different directions of gaze.

The angle of squint varies in different directions of gaze for a ____________ esotrope.

515. (1) medial recti
(2) down

516. Since the medial rectus muscle is moved down so that it is weakened in downward gaze, the rule can be formulated: **to weaken a recti muscle in a specific vertical field of gaze, move its insertion toward that field of gaze.** To weaken the lateral recti in the superior field of gaze (as in a **V** exotropia), you would move the (1) ____________ (muscle)

(2) ____________ (what direction).

663. The earlier it is treated, the better the prognosis (or equivalent wording).

664. The prognosis for restoring vision in amblyopia seems better if treatment is started before age 12.

Given cases of amblyopia in children of 5, 15, and 25 years of age, which one has the best prognosis?

811. the medial rectus contracted maximally

812. In a large esotropia, the medial rectus is contracted almost maximally. Therefore, a 4 mm recession will have a greater effect here than in a small esotropia.

Will a 4 mm recession of the medial rectus have a greater effect in a $60^{\triangle}$ ET or in a $30^{\triangle}$ ET?

69. apex

70. Prisms always displace images in the direction of the ________ .

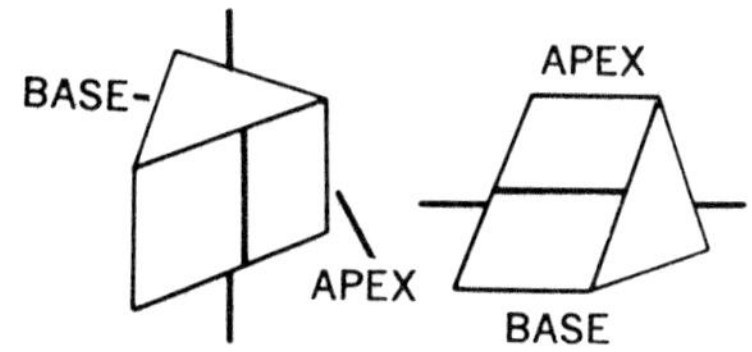

218. fuse (or integrate)

219. The terms fusion or unification are used to describe the brain's process of receiving and integrating the image information from both eyes. The brain takes the slightly different information and creates a richer impression than the image on a single retina.

Fusion is the process of (1) ________ , resulting in (2) (more/less) information to the brain than either retinal image.

367. noncomitant

368. If one of the muscles that moves the eye in a particular direction isn't working properly, that eye has difficulty moving in that particular direction. Such a muscle is called a paretic muscle.

An eye with a ________ muscle has difficulty looking in the direction of action of that muscle.

516. (1) lateral recti
(2) up

517. The theoretical basis for moving the medial rectus down is that in downward gaze the lower the muscle insertion is located, the greater the backward movement of this muscle in downward gaze. If the muscle is moved from *A* to *B*, and the eye looks down, the muscle insertion will be (according to diagram) ____________ distance farther back. Thus, the muscle will be weaker on downward gaze.

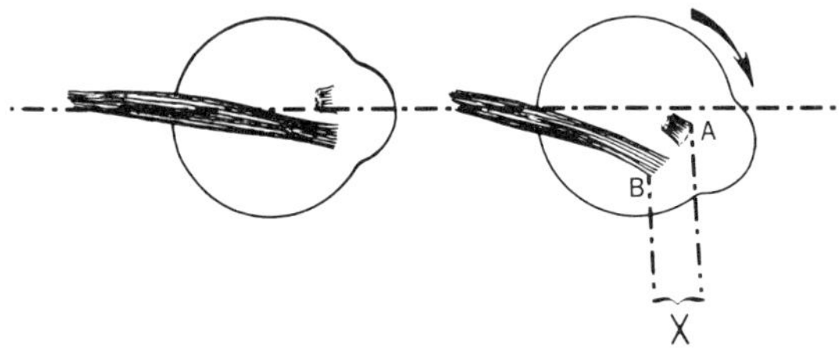

664. the five-year old

665. The newborn infant does not have the anatomical potential for 20/20 vision, but precisely how well such an infant can see is difficult to assay. We can be reasonably confident that a one-month old child can see 20/60, a one-year old 20/50 and a three-year old 20/30. Is it reasonable to believe that a five-year old child should see 20/20?

812. 60△ ET

813. In a small ET, the medial rectus is contracted only slightly more than normal. Therefore, a 6 mm recession will have less effect on its amplitude of contraction than in a large esotropia.

Since the larger the squint, the greater the effect from the same operation, would you expect some surgeons to logically perform the same recession operation on both a small and a large squint?

70. apex

71. Since prisms bend light rays, a prism can be described by designating the amount by which it bends a ray of light.

In the illustration, the ray coming from the left is bent (1) ______°. The prism could therefore be described as a (2) ______° prism.

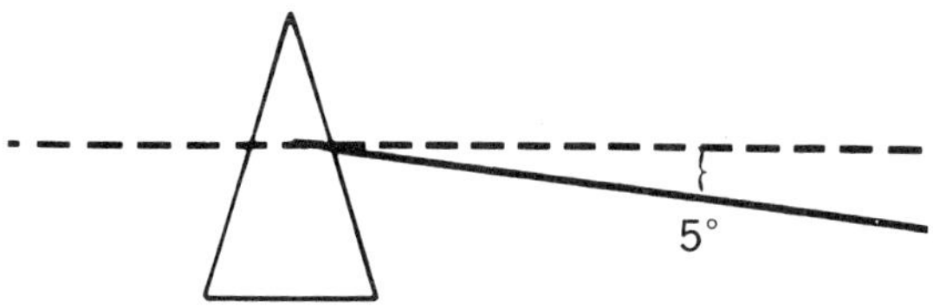

219. (1) integrating (or unificating) the image information from both eyes
(2) more

220. A stereoscope, a form of a diploscope, is any device which is so designed that separate targets may be presented simultaneously to both eyes. If the targets are properly designed, the patient should be able to appreciate depth or three dimensions when looking in a ______ .

368. paretic

369. It may be difficult to discover the presence of a paretic eye muscle if you test that eye only and keep the other eye covered. It is only by testing the movements of both eyes at the same time that you may notice that one eye does not move as well as the other.

It is usually by comparing the movement of both eyes that a ______ muscle may be discovered.

517. X

518. To weaken the medial rectus muscle in downward gaze you should ______________ .

---

665. yes

666. In alternating squints, each eye fixates on a part-time basis. Therefore, each eye gets an opportunity to be used.

Does one eye suppress vision all the time in an alternating squint?

---

813. yes

814. In a recession-resection operation for ET, the medial rectus is weakened and the lateral rectus is strengthened.

Often for an ET, the (1) ______________ is recessed and the (2) ______________ is resected.

71. (1) 5
(2) 5

72. In eye work, however, instead of describing a prism by the number of degrees it bends a ray of light, we describe a prism's strength in terms of the number of cm it displaces a ray on a screen. The actual displacement of a ray in cm will depend on where the screen is placed.

In the illustration, is the light ray displacement greatest at screen *A*, *B*, *C*, or *D*?

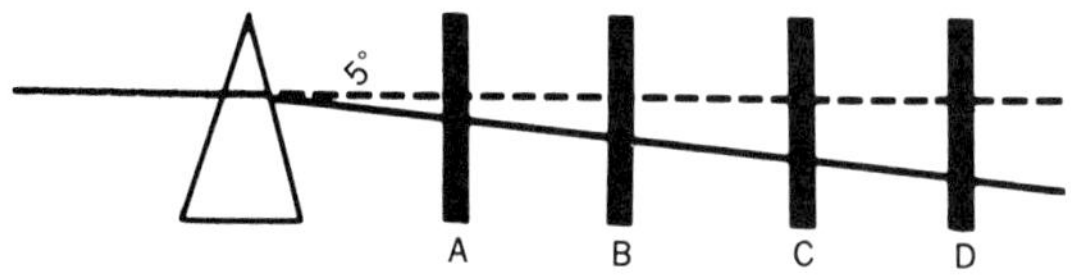

220. stereoscope

221. The ability to blend the impressions of both eyes into a single impression (fusion) has been arbitrarily graded using different types of targets in a stereoscope.

The grades of fusion have been designated in the artificial environment of the ____________ .

369. paretic

370. Noncomitant esotropia is caused by a weakness of a muscle of one eye. Therefore, if the patient looks in the direction in which the weak muscle should be working, the good eye looks at the target and the paretic eye fails to reach it. In other directions of gaze, the paretic eye is in close alignment with the good eye.

In noncomitant esotropia, the misalignment of the eyes is greatest in the field of action of the ____________ muscle.

518. move the insertion of the medial rectus down

519. Divergence excess in the superior field of gaze is usually attributed to the lateral rectus muscles. In a **V** exotrope, you might incriminate the ____________ muscles as overacting when the patient looks up (in addition to overaction or underaction of the obliques).

---

666. no

667. In an intermittent squint, both eyes sometimes appear straight and fixate simultaneously.

In an intermittent squint, does the deviating eye suppress vision at all times?

---

814. (1) medial rectus
(2) lateral rectus

815. The recession-resection operation attempts to mechanically reposition the eyeball temporally as if the muscles were strings. That is, the medial rectus is slackened and the lateral rectus ____________ .

72. *D*

73. In eye work, we assume the screen is placed 1 meter from the prism. One prism diopter (1△) deviates parallel rays of light 1 cm at 1 meter behind the prism. Therefore, a prism of 2△ strength deviates a straight ray 2 cm on a screen 1 meter away.

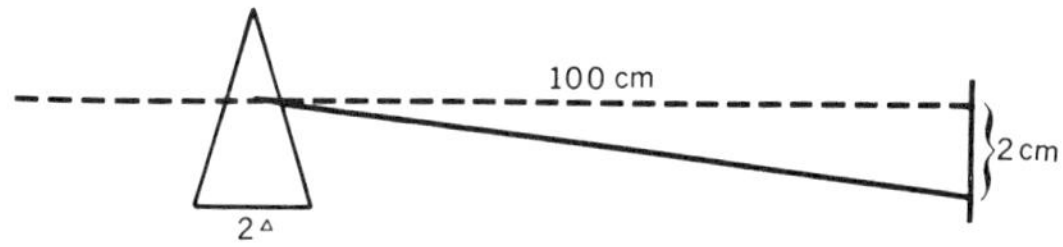

What size prism displaces a light ray 4 cm on a screen 1 meter away?

---

221. stereoscope

222. The grade of fusion is determined by the degree of precision in placing and interpreting the targets presented to each eye on corresponding areas of each retina.

The higher the level of fusion the better the eyes can place images of the targets on ____________ retinal areas.

---

370. paretic

371. In noncomitant squint, the angle of squint varies with different positions of gaze.

In noncomitant squint the angle of squint is (1) ____________ in the field of action of the paretic muscle and (2) ____________ in other fields of gaze.

519. lateral rectus

520. If the horizontal squint is large and the accompanying **A** or **V** pattern is the lesser component, the horizontal squint can be treated by itself, for the **A** or **V** pattern may resolve as the basic squint is alleviated. A patient who has a large exotropia in all fields of gaze but has a moderate **V** pattern could be reasonably treated as you would an exotrope (with/without) a **V**.

---

667. no

668. Amblyopia is generally not associated with intermittent squints or alternating squints. Two types of squints usually not associated with amblyopia are (1) __________ and (2) __________ .

---

815. tightened (or shortened)

816. If the same amount of resection of the lateral rectus is made as recession of the medial rectus, then the stretch-tension relationship is not altered.

If the medial rectus is recessed 5 mm, how many mm of resection of the lateral rectus must be made so the tension-stretch is not altered?

73. 4 prism diopters

74. We can convert prism diopters into degrees, since by definition 1△ = 1 cm at 1 meter. A circle whose radius is 1 meter has a circumference (360°) of 628 cm (or△). Therefore 1△ = .573°.

A prism of 10△ would deviate light about ______°.

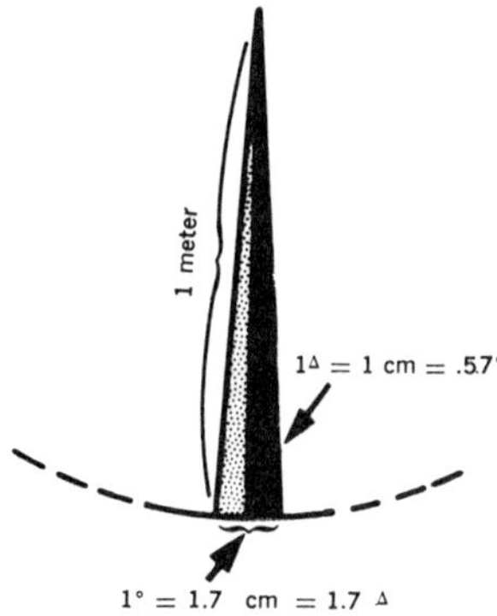

222. corresponding

223. In Grade I fusion each eye is given a dissimilar image, eg, one eye sees a lion, the other a cage.

If the patient can see the lion and the cage at the same time he is said to have ______.

371. (1) greatest
(2) less

372. The incidence of noncomitant squint is less than 1% of all squints.

Noncomitant squint is ______ compared to the incidence of comitant squint.

520. without

521. When **A** or **V** is measured, the accommodation should be controlled. This is accomplished by having the patient wear his full refractive correction and using a target which demands that accommodation be held constant, such as reasonably small letters or numbers.

To measure **A** and **V** patterns, (1) ____________ must be controlled by (2) ____________ and (3) ____________ .

668. (1) intermittent } either
(2) alternating } order

669. Depending upon the refraction in each eye, some anisometropes will use one eye for one task and the other eye for another task. A 50-year-old man with myopia of −2.00 OD and hyperopia of +1.00 OS will probably use (1) ____________ for near vision and (2) ____________ for distance vision.

816. 5

817. At present, the basic operations used for esotropia are: (a) recession of one or both medial recti, and (b) resection of one or both lateral recti in combination with (a).

The operation which should generally not be done by itself would be a ____________ of one or both lateral recti.

74. 5.73

75. The relation of prism diopters to degrees is 1.75△ = 1° or about 2△ to 1°.

If a patient has a 20△ exophoria, the exophoria is about ___________°.

223. Grade I fusion

224. In Grade II fusion testing, each eye is presented with a similar object, eg, a seal with a ball on his nose is presented to one eye and a seal with a ball on his tail is presented to the other eye. (Recall that Grade I images were dissimilar rather than similar.)

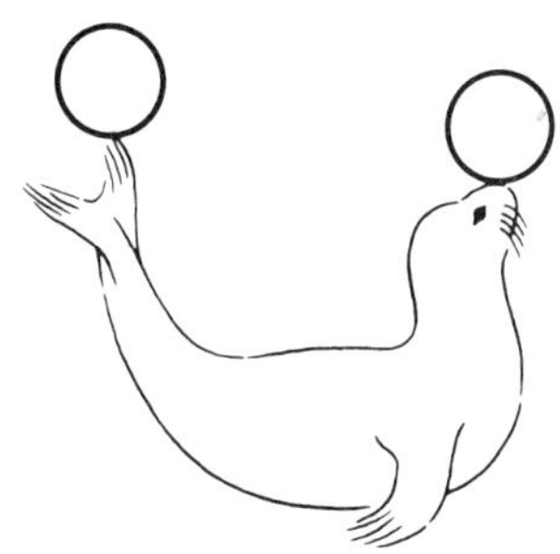

If the subject reports he sees the image diagrammed, he will also exhibit some amplitude of fusional reserve, which results from similar targets. What grade fusion does he have?

372. rare (less than 1%)

373. A rare type of noncomitant squint is called strabismus fixus. In this case, both eyes are crossed at the same time, and fixation is only possible by turning the head.

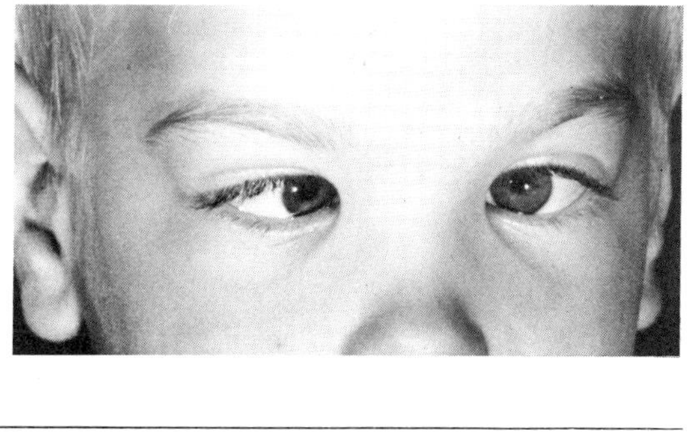

In strabismus fixus both eyes are crossed at the ___________ time.

521. (1) accommodation
(2) the full refractive correction
(3) a target which controls accommodation

(2) and (3) in either order

522. By controlling accommodation, a **V** pattern esotrope may change to have no **V** pattern, and a slight **A** pattern may become more apparent and significant. Control of accommodation (1) (increases/decreases) **V** patterns and (2) (increases/decreases) **A** patterns as compared to testing without control of accommodation.

669. (1) OD
(2) OS

670. It will be recalled that the area of the retina called the macula (the center of which is the fovea) is responsible for seeing fine details in the daytime.

Which part of the retina is best able to discriminate fine details in well lighted surroundings?

817. resection (naturally, neither should a recession)

818. There is no complete agreement as to what the indications are for each type of operation for ET. This is probably due to the fact that similar results are reported for each type of operation.

Is there universal agreement as to which type of surgery should be done for each specific type and size of esotropia?

75. 10

76. Sometimes a prism will be described in terms of degrees of displacement. A simple way to convert degrees to prism diopters is to multiply the degrees by 2.

A prism which displaces a ray 4° has a prism diopter value of approximately ________ .

224. Grade II

225. In reviewing the seal slides, we see that if each slide had a seal with a ball on the nose, the examiner couldn't tell whether the subject was fusing both slides or just seeing one seal with one eye.

Fusion slides always have controls to see that the subject ________ .

373. same

374.

PART V
VERTICAL SQUINTS

(Advance to next frame.)

522. (1) decreases
(2) increases

523. The **A** and **V** patterns which are observed when accommodation is not controlled, and which decrease as the accommodation is controlled, are termed **pseudo A** and **pseudo V** patterns. These pseudo **A** or **V** patterns (should/should not) be treated.

---

670. macula or fovea

671. The poor vision of the amblyopic eye is different from the poor vision of a diseased eye. The amblyopic eye's vision does not decrease in reduced illumination, whereas the diseased eye has disproportionately decreased vision in low illumination. If a patient has a vision of 20/200 in an eye with retinal disease, and a vision of 20/200 in the other eye that is amblyopic, which eye would function better at night?

---

818. no

819. The medial rectus inserts in front of the equator of the eyeball. If the medial rectus is recessed behind the equator, the eye loses its power to turn fully toward the nose and retracts instead.

How many mm represents a rational limit for recessing the medial rectus? (*See diagram.*)

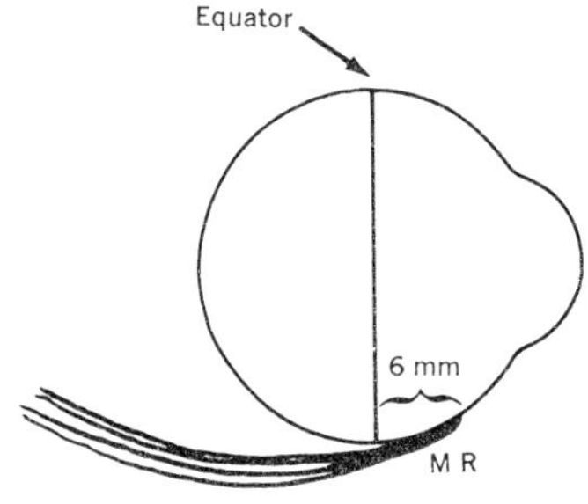

76. 8

77. If we know the value of a prism in prism diopters, we divide by 2 to get approximate degrees of displacement. A 10 prism diopter prism will displace an image approximately ____________ degrees.

225. is using both eyes

226. In Grade II fusion, not only does each eye report to the brain at the same time, but corresponding parts of each retina receive the same image. If noncorresponding parts of each retina receive images of the seals, and both report to the brain, then the patient might say that he sees two seals.

Double vision occurs when the same target is received on ____________ parts of each retina.

374. *(Advance to next frame.)*

375. Vertical ocular deviations are less common than horizontal deviations, but many horizontal squints also have a small vertical component to the deviation.

Esotropes and exotropes frequently have a moderate ____________ deviation.

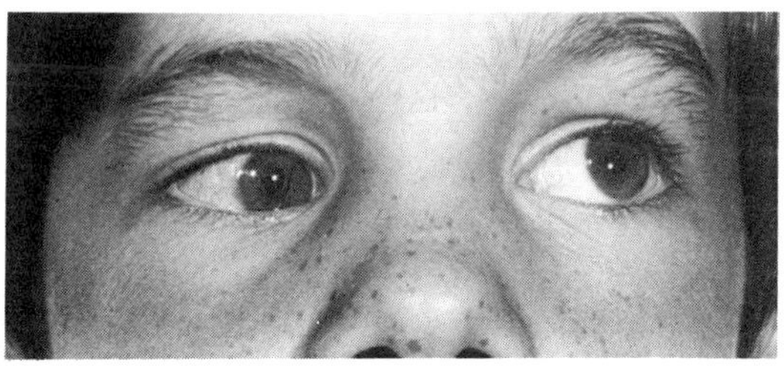

523. should not

524.

PART VII
PROGNOSIS

(Advance to next frame.)

671. the amblyopic eye

672. The amblyopic eye is a little less sensitive in appreciating that a rapidly flickering light is actually flickering and not steady.

If a normal eye can tell that a light going on and off 24 times a second is flickering, would you expect an amblyopic eye to notice a flicker at a higher or lower rate than 24 times per second?

819. 6

820. Since the success rates for the major types of muscle surgery for ET are similar, we will simply note the advantages of each method.

How do the success rates for various types of muscle surgery for ET compare?

77. 5

78. If a patient is said to have a 20° exotropia, it would be equivalent to a 40 prism diopter squint.

If a patient has a 50 prism diopter exotropia, what would that be equivalent to in degrees?

226. noncorresponding

227. The subject having Grade III fusion reports a sensation of three-dimensionality when presented with the appropriate slides. Such slides, called stereograms, present each eye with a slightly different view of the same object. The ability to fuse two stereograms and describe the sensation of depth when looking at the slides is present in ____________.

375. vertical

376. If an eye deviates up, it is called a **hypertropia**; if it deviates down, a **hypotropia**.

A right hypertropia indicates the right eye deviates ____________.

524. *(Advance to next frame.)*

525. In discussing the prognosis of our present treatment of squints, we use two criteria of success.

The first evaluates the cosmetic appearance and is easier to attain than the second. The second criterion evaluates the patients' ability to align their visual axes and fuse the retinal images.

Which criterion is easier to meet with treatment?

---

672. lower

673. An amblyopic eye cannot follow a quickly moving target as accurately as a normal eye in daylight. Why would you not expect a patient, forced to use his amblyopic eye, to gauge a good return of a fast moving tennis ball, although he can be forced to use the same eye to direct a hammer accurately on a nail?

---

820. similar

821. Generally, a significant amount of scarring is involved in the healing process after eye muscle surgery.

Analysis of previous unsuccessful squint surgery includes an estimate of the __________ resulting from the previous surgery.

78. 25 degrees

79. As a squinting patient is alternately occluded, the eyes are seen to move with each occlusion, and the patient notes a jump of the fixation target. When prisms equaling the squint are in front of the patient, there will be (1) (no/some) movement of the eyes with alternate occlusions, and the patient will report (2) (no/some) movement of the target with each alternate occlusion.

227. Grade III fusion

228. In Grade III fusion, the retinal images fall partially on corresponding areas and partially on noncorresponding areas. A high degree of precision is needed to align the images.

For a stereoscopic effect each retinal image falls on (1) ____________ and (2) ____________ parts of each retina.

376. up

377. Although hypotropia means that an eye deviates down, it is customary to describe a vertical deviation by denoting which eye deviates up, ie, in terms of hypertropia. The eyes are so related that a vertical deviation can be described either as a left hypotropia or a right hypertropia. A right hypotropia can also be referred to as a ____________ .

525. cosmetic

526. The cosmetic correction of a squint is a major success. This enables the previously disfigured child to be accepted as a normal member of his family and society and to enjoy the accompanying advantages.

How may a squint be a contribution to maladjustment of a child?

673. Because the amblyopic eye follows a fast moving target poorly (or equivalent words).

674. The amblyopic eye will often not be able to read a line of letters, but will be able to identify the letters if presented one at a time.

Would you expect visual acuity in an amblyopic eye to be better if single letters or lines of letters are used for testing?

821. scars (or adhesions)

822. Often, an increased amount of scar tissue forms if there has been a great deal of bleeding during the surgery.

The amount of ____________ during surgery appears to be directly proportional to the development of scar formation after surgery.

79. (1) no
(2) no

80. Prisms are a convenient method of effectively changing the fixation object when alternately occluding the eyes. If prisms base-out, of increasing amounts, are placed before an esotropic eye and the eyes alternately occluded, the eyes will move less and less as more prism is added. When the prism power equals the esotropia, ____________ movement will be seen as the eyes are alternately occluded.

228. (1) corresponding } either
(2) noncorresponding } order

229. The stereoscope is not the only way to test for fusion. However, in each method a target is presented to each eye with a control so that the examiner knows which eye sees which target. In the picture, OS is looking at a clock. A small mirror is placed in front of OD for two reasons. It does not allow OD to see the clock, but it does allow OD to see a light. If the subject has Grade I fusion, what should he see? (*Refer to the diagram.*)

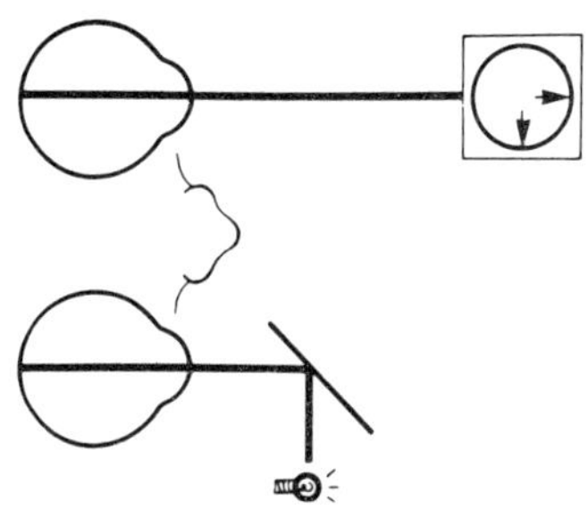

377. left hypertropia

378. A left hypertropia is the same, in effect, as a right hypotropia, and a left hypotropia is the same as a ____________ . Remember that vertical squints are usually described in terms of the hypertropic eye.

526. Such a child is not cosmetically acceptable by family or society. (or similar words)

527. If treatment of a squint established a normal type of fusion of both retinal images by the brain, the patient's visual world would become richer and in certain situations permit him to perceive three-dimensionality.

In a situation devoid of clues except for the retinal disparity, such as looking from a plane,

(1) Could a subject with normal fusion appreciate three-dimensionality? __________
(2) Could a patient with squint appreciate three-dimensionality? __________

---

674. single letters

675. The amblyope's inability to discriminate letters which are close together (crowded together) as well as he can discriminate isolated letters is referred to as the phenomenon of crowding.

The patient who can read 20/70 in a chart, but can read 20/40 when isolated letters are shown, demonstrates the phenomenon of __________ .

---

822. bleeding

823. Increased scar formation may also result from an increased body response to some forms of suture material which act as a foreign substance. For example, nonabsorbable suture induces less reaction around it than catgut.

Would you expect more scar formation after surgery involving nonabsorbable or catgut?

80. no

81. As the cover is switched from OD to OS, the center of the cornea moves from *A* to *B*, indicating that the patient has ____________ tropia.

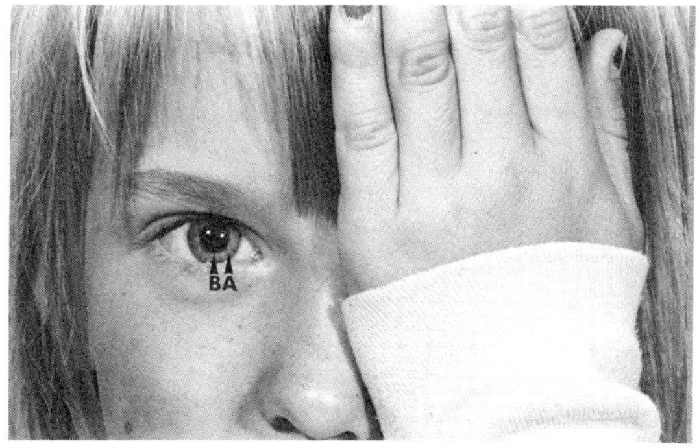

229. The light superimposed on the clock. 

230. The subject in the picture has a red glass before one eye and a green glass before the other and is looking at a white light. What does OD see? (1) ____________ What does OS see? (2) ____________

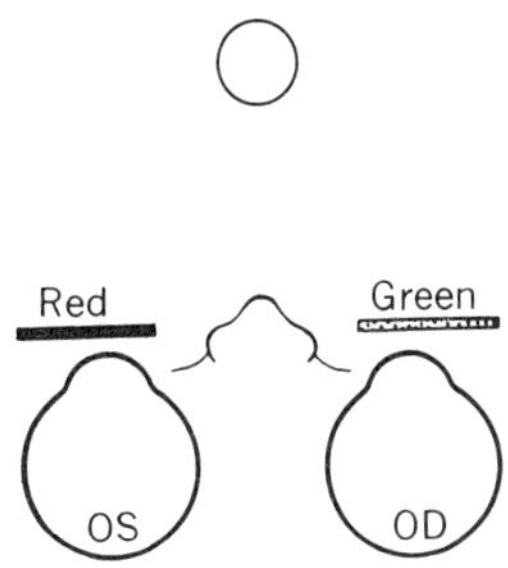

378. right hypertropia

379. A vertical squint is measured in the same fashion as a horizontal squint; that is, either by estimation of the corneal reflexes or by alternate occlusion accompanied by neutralization of eye motions with prisms.

Vertical squints are measured the same way as ____________ .

527. (1) yes
(2) no

528. A cosmetic success is defined as one in which the angle of squint after treatment is less than 15 prism diopters.

Would a case that had 60 prism diopters of esotropia before treatment and 25 prism diopters of esotropia after treatment be considered a success? (1) ____________ (2) Why?

---

675. crowding

676. Identical twins who have similar squints have been followed for several years. One twin may develop amblyopia, although his twin may have an identical squint, and not develop amblyopia.

From the above, we can say that the amblyopia associated with squints probably (is/is not) inherited.

---

823. catgut

824. Scar formation is the body's method of cementing cut ends of tissue together; therefore, it is indispensable to the success of surgery.

In a recession of the medial rectus, the formation of ____________ unites the muscle to its new position on the eyeball.

81. eso

82. With the fixating eye covered, the visual axis of the deviated eye rotates to fixate the target. Therefore, to measure the angle of the squint, all we do is cover the fixating eye and measure how much the deviating eye turns to pick up fixation.

In almost all squints, if the fixating eye is covered, the deviating eye turns to pick up fixation. This amount of turn is equal to the ______________ .

---

230. (1) a green light
(2) a red light

231. The subject in the diagram has Grade II fusion, and the images fall on corresponding parts of the retinas. He will report the single light as a reddish-green light. A reddish-green light from a patient indicates he is using (the right/the left/both) retina(s).

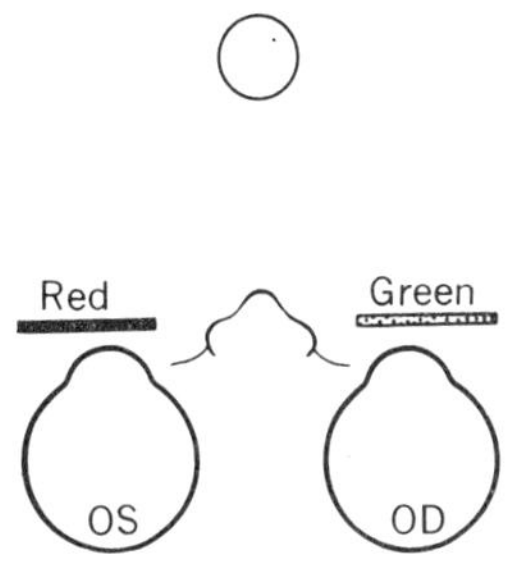

---

379. horizontal squints

380. If the corneal reflex on the right eye is 1 mm below the center of the right pupil as compared to the corresponding reflex on the left eye, the patient has (1) ______________ △ right hypertropia. (1 mm = 7.5° or 15△)

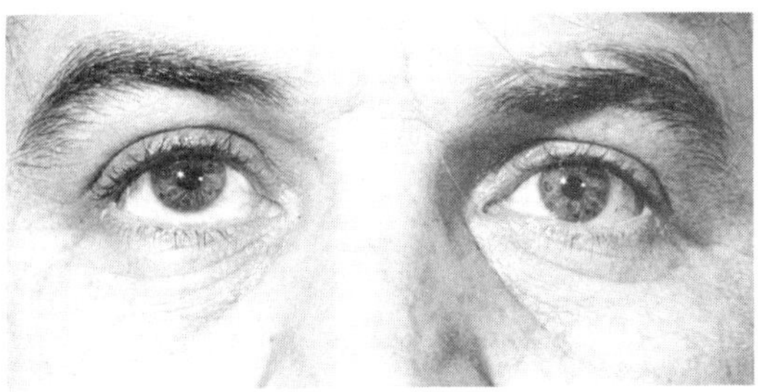

528. (1) no
(2) The residual squint is greater than 15 prism diopters (cosmetically unacceptable).

529. Success of treatment in terms of fusion is often divided into the level or degree of fusion attained. Fewer patients attain third degree fusion (stereopsis) than first degree (simultaneous perception) or second degree (fusion of similar images).

(A) Is the attainment of stereopsis after squint treatment as common as the attainment of simultaneous perception of retinal images?

(B) List the grades of fusion in order of their frequency of attainment after squint surgery.

---

676. is not

677. A different pattern of brain wave electrical activity is often recorded when the amblyopic eye looks at something and when the normal eye looks at the same thing.

Does stimulation of an amblyopic eye induce brain wave activity similar to or different from one induced when a normal eye is stimulated?

---

824. scar tissue

825. When a reoperation is indicated because the original surgery resulted in an overcorrection or undercorrection, the job is technically more difficult if a great deal of scar formation is present.

The presence of ____________ makes the reoperation more difficult.

82. angle of squint

83. To measure the size of a squint, cover the fixating eye, forcing the other to turn to pick up fixation. Now, start placing prisms before the fixating eye while intermittently occluding that eye. When a prism equal to the amount of squint is placed before the fixating eye, as the cover is removed from that eye, neither eye will move. This is called the **cover test with prisms**. The strength of the prism used in the cover test is a measure of __________ .

231. both

232. The subject in the diagram has the eyes misaligned so that the images from the light fall on noncorresponding retinal points. He will report that he simultaneously sees a (1) __________ light and a (2) __________ light.

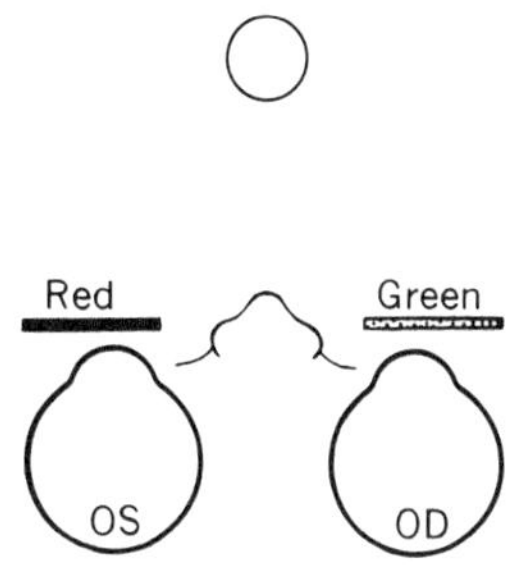

380. 15

381. If the corneal reflex on the left cornea is 1½ mm below the center of the left cornea as compared to the corresponding reflex on the right cornea, the patient has (1) __________ Δ (2) __________ hypertropia.

529. (A) no
(B) (1) first degree
(2) second degree
(3) third degree

530. In order to best evaluate the improvement of a squint attributed to a special treatment, one should know what improvement to expect if no treatment is administered.

What is wrong with this statement?—Since the patient's squint improved after drinking snake oil for 4 weeks, the snake oil must have been responsible for the improvement.

---

677. different

678. The phenomenon of crowding exhibited by an amblyope demonstrates that the optics, fovea, and neural pathways are capable of functioning at a level better than indicated on chart testing. This implies that the optics, fovea, and neural pathway to the brain of an amblyope (are/are not) responsible for the reduced vision.

---

825. scar tissue

826. If the area of insertion of a muscle is obscured and covered by a great deal of scar tissue, isolation of the muscle and subsequent relocation of the muscle is surgically difficult and not precise.

A great deal of scar tissue covering a muscle insertion interferes with ____________ of the muscle and its subsequent relocation.

83. the angle of squint

84. The measurement of an exotropia with the cover test utilizes base- ____________ prisms to neutralize eye movements.

232. (1) red } either
(2) green } order

233. It is known that with a green lens placed before the eye, a green light can be seen, but a red light is invisible. Conversely, with a red lens before the eye, a (1) ____________ light can be seen, but a (2) ____________ light is invisible.

381. (1) 22.5
(2) left

382. This patient has a ____________ hypertropia.

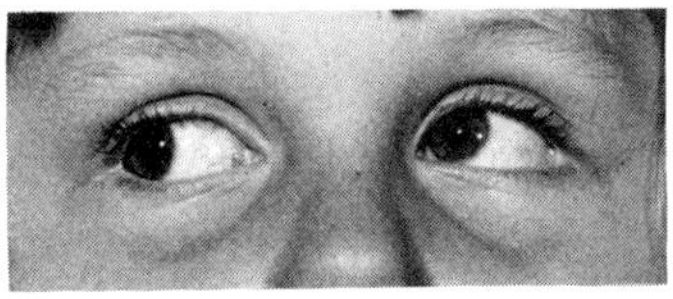

530. The squint might have improved with no treatment.

531. In a series of 122 children with constant esotropia (the majority being of the nonaccommodative type) followed without treatment for an average of 10 years, about 50% showed no change in the size of the squint.

Of 1000 four-year-old children, each with an esotropia of 60 prism diopters, about how many would still have a 60 prism diopter esotropia at age 14?

---

678. are not

679. If brain wave activity is different when the amblyopic eye is stimulated, we must assume that either the signal from the retina is different or the brain's activity in response to a normal signal is different or brain and retinal functions are both different.

From brain wave evidence, where is the site of disturbance in amblyopia?

---

826. isolation

827. If more surgery is indicated after a resection-recession operation on one eye, the muscles of the other eye may be operated on, thus avoiding attacking the scar formation from the first operation.

One advantage of a recession-resection operation is that the ____________ is available for further surgery.

84. in

85. When the front of the eye turns out, the back of the eye rotates in.

If the cornea turns temporally, the retina must rotate ________.

233. (1) red
(2) green

234. In the Worth 4-dot test, the subject wears a red glass over the right eye and a green glass over the left eye. He looks at the target of lights pictured. If the left eye is occluded, what does he see? ________
(draw diagram)

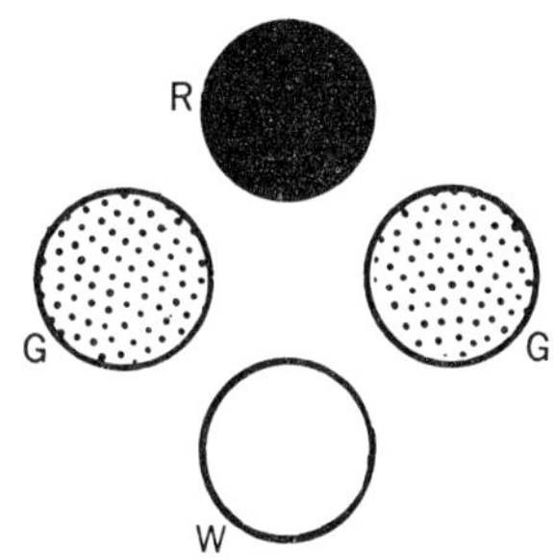

382. left

383. If alternate occlusion of a patient's eyes results in the right eye rotating down to fixate and the left eye rotating up to fixate, the patient has a ________.

531. 500

532. In the series of 122 esotropes followed for an average of 10 years, 10% showed an increase in the size of their squint, and about 40% showed a decrease in their angle of squint.

In a group of 100 young esotropes, given no therapy, (1) ________ (number) will improve, (2) ________ (number) will get worse, and (3) ________ (number) will stay the same.

---

679. either brain, retina, or both

680. Experiments on newborn kittens who were made to wear a diffusing screen (similar to bathroom window glass) over one eye for three months indicate that an abnormality develops in the cells of the visual cortex associated with that eye.

If form vision is not allowed to develop in kittens, where in the visual system does an abnormality occur?

---

827. other eye

828. After a recession-resection operation on one eye, the eye may be bandaged without interfering with vision. Naturally, bandaging both eyes after surgery incapacitates and frightens the patient.

Bandaging one operated eye after uniocular surgery is not incapacitating. Generally, we (should/should not) bandage both eyes even if we do binocular surgery.

85. nasally

86. In the case of exotropia, if the fixating eye were covered and a base-in prism of correct strength were placed in front of the deviating eye, the deviating eye would not have to turn in to pick up fixation, because the prism bends the rays so that they fall on the fovea. In the illustration, a base- (1) ____________ prism is used to get the image on the fovea of an eye which is turned (2) ____________ .

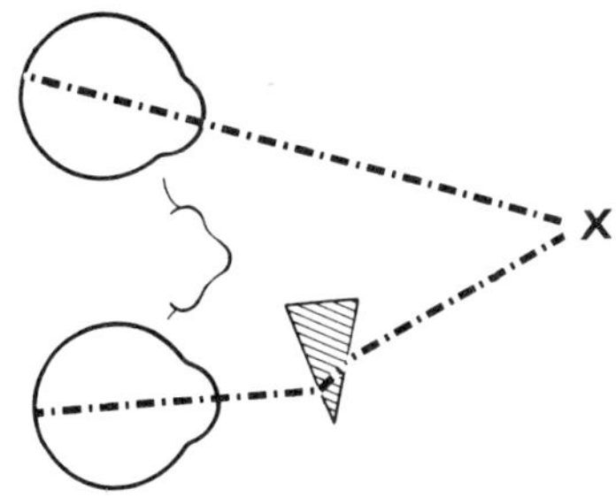

234. R ●
R ●

235. Again using the Worth 4-dot test with the subject having a red glass over OD and a green glass over OS, he looks at the dots.

If the right eye is occluded, what does he see?

____
(draw diagram)

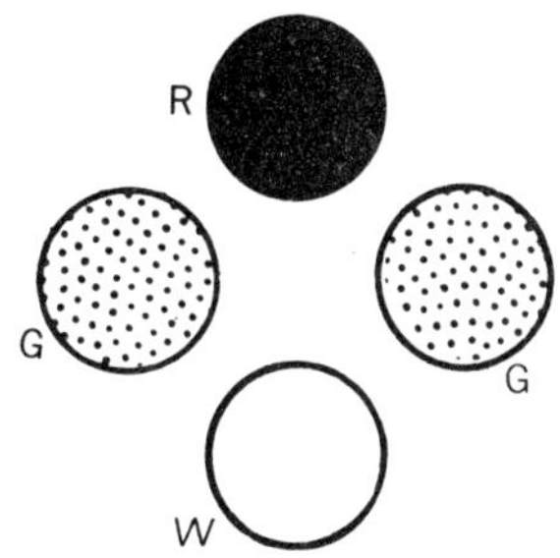

383. right hypertropia

384. If alternate occlusion results in the right eye rotating up to fixate and the left eye rotating down to fixate, the patient has a ____________ .

532. (1) 40
(2) 10
(3) 50

533. Although about 40% of the series of young esotropes improved, only 15% improved enough to be considered cosmetically straight, and only one child developed fusion.

If not given any treatment, how many young esotropes in a group of 100 will probably look cosmetically straight after ten years?

---

680. visual cortex (or brain)

681. Although it is not always correct to assume that what is true in lower animals is true in humans, we may guess from the kitten experiment that the site of the disturbance in amblyopia is in the visual cortex.

From present evidence in kittens, where would you guess the site of difficulty lies in amblyopia?

---

828. should not

829. The advantages of a uniocular recession-resection operation also apply to a uniocular recession alone. Both give greater freedom to the surgeon if a ___________ is indicated.

86. (1) in
(2) out

87. In a patient with exotropia, if a 20 prism diopter prism, base-in, is needed to neutralize movement of the right eye when the left is covered, the patient is said to have 20 prism diopters of exotropia.

If a 30 prism diopter prism neutralized one-half the movement of the deviating eye during the cover test, how large is the squint?

235. 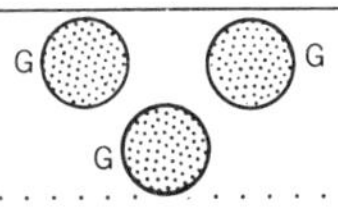

236. The subject has a red glass over OD and a green glass over OS and looks at the Worth 4-dot test. If he has normal fusion, he will see ________ .

(draw diagram)

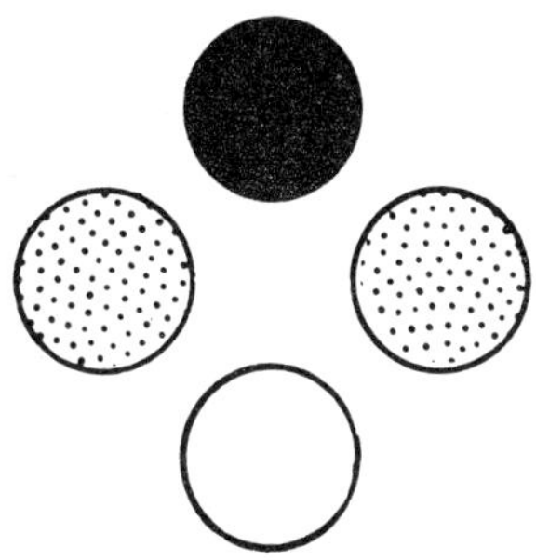

384. left hypertropia

385. Prisms point relatively the same way for measuring vertical squints as they do for measuring horizontal squints. The apex points in the direction of the squint (ie, apex points in for esotrope and out for exotrope). Prism base-up OD (apex points down OD) measures a right hypotropia (left hypertropia). Prism base-down OD (apex points up OD) measures a ________ .

533. 15

534. In a similar study in which twenty-six young intermittent esotropes were followed for an average of eight years, almost one-half of the cases achieved constant straight eyes and fusion.

What percentage of a group of five-year-old intermittent esotropes would you predict to outgrow the condition?

681. visual cortex

682. Not only does the fovea need a distinct image in order that it develop properly and avoid amblyopia, but the image must be in focus in all meridions. If a child has simple myopic astigmatism with only the 90° meridion in focus on the fovea, a specific inability to see clearly in the 180° meridion can be demonstrated to persist in adulthood when the optical defect was later corrected. Meridional amblyopia implies defective vision in (specific/all) meridions.

829. reoperation

830. The major advantage of recession of both medial recti for ET is that both eyes are affected equally by the surgery and so move symmetrically in the various positions of gaze.

Would a bimedial recession or a uniocular recession-resection be more likely to cause asymmetrical eye movement in various positions of gaze?

87. 60 prism diopters

88. If an eye turns out, the fovea turns nasally. Therefore, base-in prism bends the rays toward the fovea in an exotropic eye.

Are base-in or base-out prisms used to neutralize exotropia?

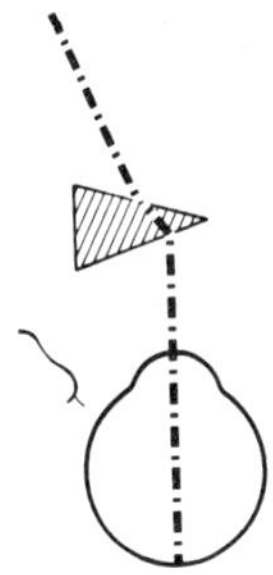

236. 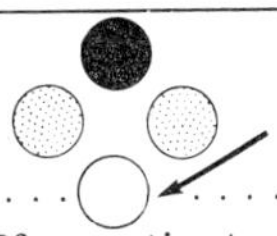 This dot will be reported red, green, or reddish-green.

237. If a patient cannot fuse the images of both eyes, he either reports double vision or he erases from his mind the report of an image from one eye.

If a subject cannot fuse, he either reports ____________ or he suppresses one image.

385. right hypertropia

386. Prism base-down OD or prism base-____________ OS will measure a right hypertropia.

534. 40 to 50%

535. The prognosis in early exotropia without treatment is different from esotropia. Although no figures are available, few cases get better. Generally, the best one can hope for is an arrest in the progress of exotropia.

If no treatment is given, is the prognosis better in esotropia or exotropia?

---

682. specific

683. Although the part of the visual cortex which represents the fovea of the amblyopic eye is not functioning properly in amblyopia, most amblyopes will direct the foveal area to a fixation target.

On what part of the retina do most amblyopes attempt to place a retinal image?

---

830. uniocular recession-resection

831. Incomitancy refers to the eyes showing different angles of squint as they look in various directions. Incomitancy is greater after uniocular surgery than after bimedial recession surgery.

The residual squint after bimedial recession surgery on an originally comitant squint would be less, but still ____________ in all positions of gaze.

88. base-in

89. Prisms placed base temporally are called base-out prisms and place the image on the fovea of an eye which has deviated ________.

237. double vision (diplopia)

238. When the red glass is before an eye that suppresses vision, no red light is seen.

If OD is suppressed and a green glass is before OS, what does the patient see? (*diagram*)

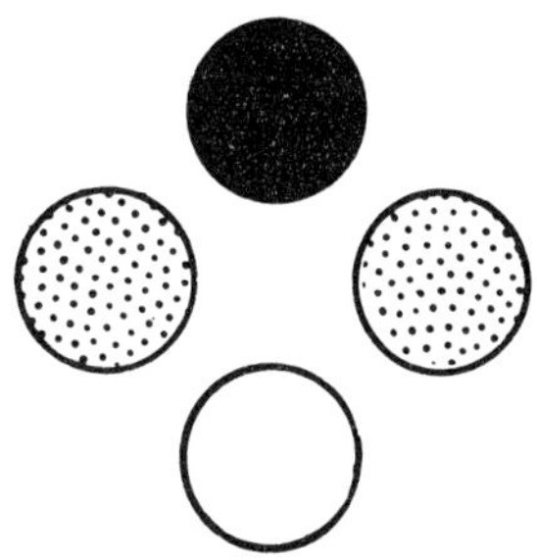

386. up

387. Since the correcting prism points in the direction of the squint, prism base-down OD corrects a right hypertropia, and prism base-up OS corrects a ________.

535. esotropia

536. The accommodative type of esotropia has a better prognosis than other types. In the accommodative type of esotropia, which becomes straight and fuses with glasses, most will be able to retain their straight eyes without their glasses by the time they become teenagers if their hyperopia is less than 2.50 D.

If a child with a fully accommodative esotropia with hyperopia of 2.50 D asks you if he will always have to wear glasses, what would you answer?

683. fovea

684. When an amblyope loses or never develops the ability to direct his fovea toward a fixation target, he will fixate eccentrically to the fovea and is called a(n) ____________ fixator.

831. comitant (or the same)

832. If a patient who has had squint surgery fuses when looking straight ahead, but has a residual squint when he looks up and to the right, then his newly gained fusion is constantly being interrupted in certain positions of gaze. Some investigators feel that eventually the patient may lose the ability to ____________ in the straight ahead position and redevelop a squint. In recent years, fewer and fewer surgeons ascribe to this line of reasoning and believe a good surgical recess-resect does not produce significant incomitancy.

89. in (or nasally)

90. Base-in prisms give a measurement of (1) ________________. Base-out prisms measure (2) ________________.

238. 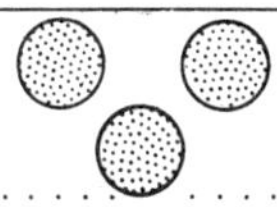

239. If a subject has a squint and doesn't suppress the impression of one eye, he reports diplopia. If a patient has diplopia, what will each eye see when viewing the Worth dots while wearing the red-green glasses? (1) Sketch. (2) How many total lights will he report?

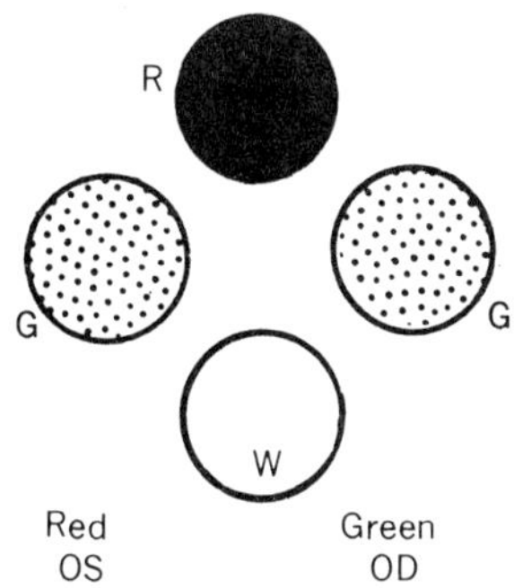

387. right hypertropia

388. Prism base-down OS or prism base-________________ OD will measure a left hypertropia.

536. The chances are good that he will not have to wear them as a teenager or thereafter.

537. It must be recalled that *fully* accommodative esotropes belong to a small minority within the classification of esotropia, but all esotropes probably have an accommodative component.

What is the effect of correcting a refractive error in a patient with a partially accommodative esotropia?

---

684. eccentric

685. A very small number of amblyopes, about ________ %, become eccentric fixators.

(See Table 1 preceding the index.)

---

832. fuse

833. Most principles of surgery for ET are applicable in surgery for XT; however, a recession for an XT involves the (1)________ rectus muscle, and a resection for an XT involves the (2)________ rectus muscle.

90. (1) exotropia
(2) esotropia

91. Exotropia is measured with (1) ____________ prisms. Esotropia is measured with (2) ____________ prisms.

239. (1) 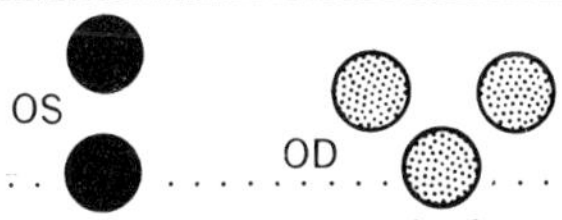

(2) 5

240. It must be remembered that there is not always a correlation between the grade of fusion demonstrated in the stereoscope and the way a patient sees the real world.

Could an occasional patient have only Grade I fusion in the stereoscope, yet appreciate three-dimensionality in the real world?

388. up

389. Placing 3^{Δ} base-up over OD has the same effect as placing 3^{Δ} base-down over OS. 6^{Δ} base-down OD gives the same effect as (1) ____________ $^{\Delta}$ base- (2) ____________ OS.

537. The angle of squint decreases.

538. Although there is no tight relationship between the age the esotropia first appears and the prognosis, it is felt that if a squint is present at birth, the prognosis for fusion development is poor.

What is the prognosis in a case of congenital esotropia?

685. 2

686. An eccentric fixator will have the retinal image of the fixation point at some point on the retina other than the fovea.

Of all the areas on the retina that an eccentric fixator might choose to place a retinal image, where would he never put the image?

833. (1) lateral
(2) medial

834. A number of controlled studies indicate a significantly higher success rate for the unilateral recession-resection operation in XT over the other possible operations.

In general, the ____________ operation has the best prognosis in XT.

91. (1) base-in
(2) base-out

92. As occlusion is rapidly alternated while the squinting patient fixates on one object, the eyes rapidly move. When this movement is neutralized by the appropriate prism, the squint is measured. If a 25 prism diopter prism base-out neutralizes the movement of the eyes with alternate occlusion, the patient has (1) ______ (2) ______ .
(amount) (type squint)

240. yes

241. Diplopia or double vision results when both visual axes are not pointing at the same object, as in a squint when no suppression exists. Under such circumstances, the image of the object appears on the fovea of the fixating eye and on some noncorresponding part of the deviating eye. If OS is fixating, what point on the OD retina is stimulated by the target?

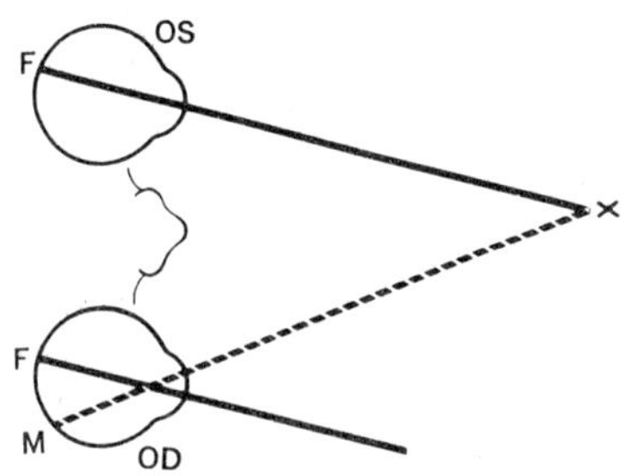

389. (1) 6
(2) up

390. If 4△ base-down OD is needed, the same effect can be obtained by 2△ base-down OD plus ______ △ base-up OS.

538. poor for fusion development

539. It has also been shown that if an esotropia first develops between the ages of three and five, appropriate treatment restores fusion in almost 80% of the cases.

Of 100 children who developed an esotropia between ages three and five, how many will demonstrate normal binocular vision after treatment?

686. fovea

687. An eccentric fixator usually attempts to place the retinal image on an inconstant area some distance from the macula. The macula of an eccentric fixator will usually be a (constant/variable) distance from the retinal image of the fixation point.

834. unilateral recession-resection

835. There is some evidence that in the case of intermittent XT of the infrequent, divergence excess variety, recessions of both lateral recti may have a slightly higher success rate than recession-resection operations of one eye.

Bilateral recessions are probably the operation of choice in a case of intermittent XT of the ____________ variety.

92. (1) 25△
(2) esotropia

93. As a squinting patient's eyes are alternately occluded and fixation is maintained on the same object, eye movement after each alternate occlusion will occur until prisms __________ to the squint are in front of the patient.

241. point *M* (on temporal retina)

242. If one eye deviates out, diplopia may result. In such an instance, the fovea of OS reports to the brain the impression of a certain target. The noncorresponding point in the OD, point *M*, reports the same impression.

The fovea of OS and point *M* of OD are considered __________ retinal areas.

390. 2

391. If 5△ base-up OD and 6△ base-down OS are used at the same time to measure a squint, the patient has (1) __________ △ (2) __________ hypertropia. (Remember that the vertical prismatic effect is the sum of prisms if base-up in one eye and base-down on the other eye.)

539. about 80

540. Unfortunately, most esotropia develops early in life, and the percentage of esotropia developing after age three would be less than 50%.

Do most cases of esotropia have their onset before or after age three?

---

687. variable

688. Since the real macula is the only retinal area anatomically constructed to detect fine detail, a false macula can never develop good acuity. Why is a false macula limited in this way?

---

835. divergence excess

836. Although determining the amount of eye muscle surgery to perform in a precise, mathematical manner is unrealistic, it appears that a recession of the lateral rectus of from 6 to 9 mm yields the best results in the recession-resection operation for XT of any amount.

Generally, a recession of (1) ____________ to (2) ____________ mm offers the best results in a recession-resection operation for XT.

93. equal

94. If the strength of the correcting prism is greater than the amount of the squint, alternate occlusion will cause the eye (of an esotrope) to move in instead of out as it is uncovered. A reversal of movement of an eye as alternate occlusion is done indicates that too <u>(much/little)</u> prism is in place.

---

242. noncorresponding

243. Corresponding retinal areas appear to have a unique quality. Each set of corresponding retinal areas is linked with a specific direction in space for each direction of the eye. If the fovea is stimulated by a target, and the eyes are straight ahead, one gets the impression of something being straight ahead.

Each pair of corresponding retinal areas has a specific ____________ .

---

391. (1) 11
(2) left

392. If 5△ base-down OD and 4△ base-up OS are needed to measure a squint, the patient has (1) ____________ △ (2) ____________ hypertropia.

540. before

541. The only other fact associated with age and prognosis has to do with the length of time the child has the squint before treatment is started. It appears that the chances of establishing single binocular vision are greater if treatment can be started less than a year after onset.

Is the prognosis for a squint whose duration is 24 months better or worse than one with a duration of six months?

---

688. It is not anatomically constructed to appreciate fine detail (or equivalent words).

689. To test whether the patient fixates centrally or eccentrically, the examiner looks at the retina with an ophthalmoscope-like device called a Visuscope.

What instrument is used to test for central fixation?

---

836. (1) 6
(2) 9

837. When muscle anomalies or abnormal adhesions are noted at surgery, preoperative plans may have to be altered. For example, in a case of medial rectus weakness, if surgical exposure reveals the medial rectus to appear normal but bound down by adhesions, simple severance of the ____________ may decrease the amount of resection necessary.

94. much

95. The patient is an esotrope. With a prism of 25△ base-out, one eye moves in as the other eye is occluded. This movement in instead of out means that the squint is (more/less) than 25△.

---

243. direction in space

244. If both eyes are looking straight ahead and a light is flashed on the left, the nasal retina of OS and the temporal retina OD are stimulated. These areas are corresponding. In the illustration, point *B* on the nasal retina OS is corresponding to a point on the ____________ of OD.

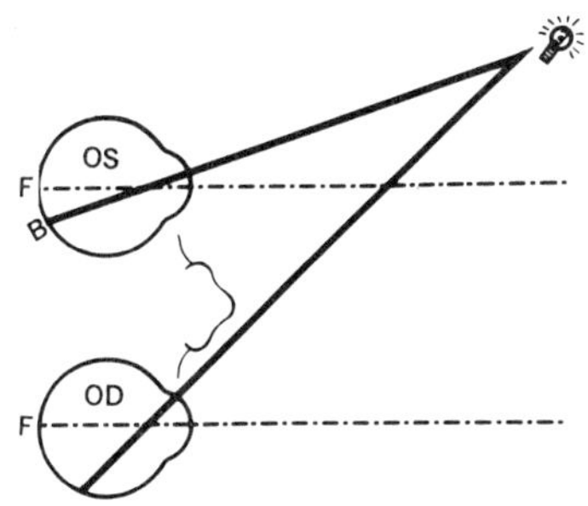

---

392. (1) 9
(2) right

393. The corneal reflexes are aligned with an 8△ prism as diagrammed. The patient has (1)____________ △ (2)____________ .

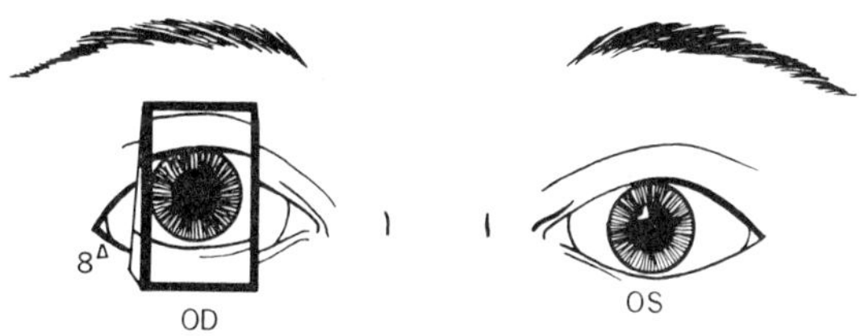

541. worse

542. The size of a constant esotropia before treatment does not affect the prognosis for fusion by any significant amount.

If you saw two cases of constant, nonaccommodative esotropia of similar age and duration, one of which measured 60 prism diopters and the other 25 prism diopters, which one would have the better prognosis?

---

689. Visuscope

690. The Visuscope not only allows the examiner to see the retina, but also projects various targets onto the retina which can be seen by both the subject and examiner. The Visuscope is a modified ophthalmoscope which ____________ onto the retina.

---

837. adhesions

838. The surgeon must be ready to alter his preoperative surgical plans if unforeseen anomalies appear at surgery.

Should an eye surgeon always follow his carefully worked out preoperative surgical plan?

95. less

96. With a prism of 15△ base-out in front of the right eye, no movement of the eye is seen when the eyes are alternately occluded. The patient has (1) ____________ (2) ____________ .
(amount) (type squint)

244. temporal retina

245. Although the subject pictured in the preceding frame is looking straight ahead, stimulation of the nasal retina OS separately or in combination with the stimulation of the temporal retina OD tells him that the light is to the left.

Points on the nasal retina OS are assigned visual direction linked to the (1) ____________ side of space.

Points on the temporal retinal OD are assigned visual direction linked to the (2) ____________ side of space.

393. (1) 8
(2) right hypertropia

394. 5△ aligns the eye in the diagram. This patient has (1) ____________ △ (2) ____________ .

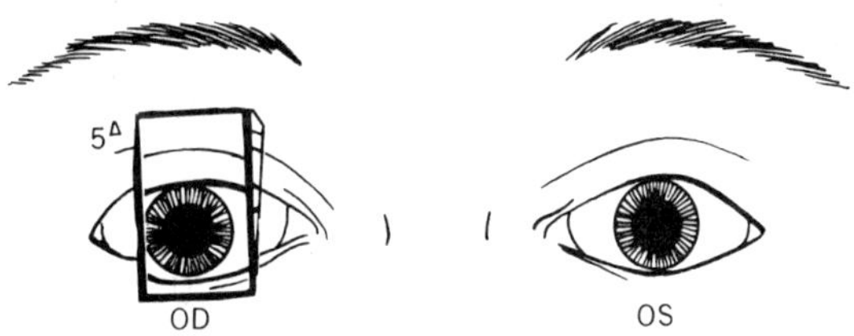

542. Both would have the same.

543. In the case of intermittent exotropia, a squint of under 20 prism diopters has a better chance for a fusional cure.

Does angle of squint affect the prognosis in constant esotropia? (1) ____________ In intermittent exotropia? (2) ____________

690. projects various targets

691. Using the Visuscope, the examiner asks the subject to look at the target projected on the retina. If the target becomes superimposed on the macula, the patient is fixating centrally. The patient in *C* is fixating on the cross. What type of fixation is he utilizing?

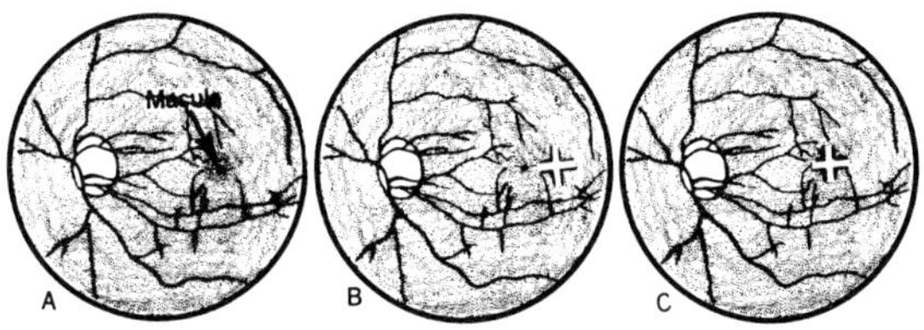

838. no

839. The conjunctiva often acts as an adhesive band. Accordingly, the conjunctiva is often recessed in reoperations, congenital strabismus, and paralytic strabismus. The bare sclera heals well and a white, quiet eye results. To achieve maximum effect of a recess-resect reoperation, a ____________ of the conjunctiva might be done on the side of the recessed muscle.

96. (1) 15$^{\triangle}$
(2) esotropia

97. By placing the proper amount of prism in front of a deviating eye, the eye will appear straight.

The strength of prism placed before a deviating eye to give the eye a straight appearance describes the ____________ of the squint.

245. (1) left
(2) left

246. If we were to put a panoramic picture of the world in front of us and break it into many small elliptical areas, we would see that with the eyes pointing toward a given spot on the picture, corresponding areas on each retina are assigned specific locations on the picture.

Therefore, if corresponding retinal areas are stimulated by a light in a darkened room, the brain knows where in space the light was flashed because each retinal area is assigned a ____________ .

394. (1) 5
(2) left hypertropia

395. Vertical squints constitute (1)____________% of all types of squint and are (2)____________% of the general population.

(See Table 1 preceding index.)

543. (1) no
(2) yes

544. Recall that in some cases of squint, by using a mirror or a prism before the deviating eye, light rays from a target can fall on the foveas of both eyes. Under these conditions fusion may occur.

What does the diagrammed patient with right esotropia see with the correcting prism if he has fusion? (*sketch*)

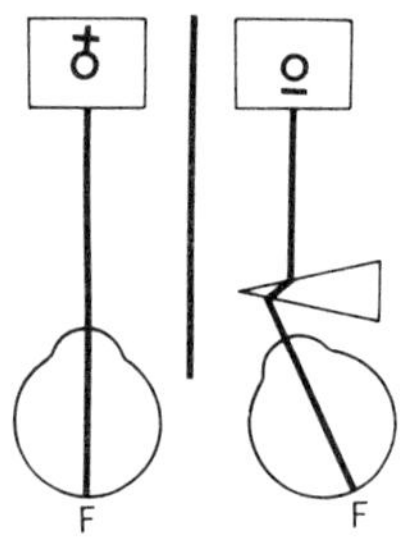

691. central fixation

692. Using the Visuscope, if the target is superimposed in an area other than the macula, then the patient is fixating eccentrically. What type of fixation is this patient using?

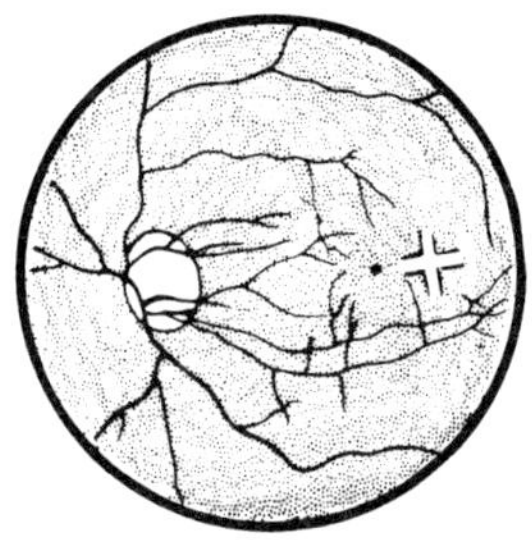

839. recession

840. A number of lessons have been learned from postoperative complications. For example, because the site of tucking often adheres to the eyeball, the muscle stretching effect of the tucking operation may be cancelled by the recession effect.

A muscle ______________ operation is unpredictable.

97. size (or amount, or angle)

98. A modification of the Hirshberg measurement is the Krimsky method. The Krimsky method centers the corneal reflex with the appropriate prism. If 25△ base-out are needed to center the corneal reflex of one eye (reflex is in center of other cornea), the patient has (1) ____________ (amount) (2) ____________ (type squint) as measured by the (3) ____________ method.

246. specific direction

247. In a patient with double vision, if the same target stimulates noncorresponding retinal areas, each stimulated retinal area reports that the target is in the locale to which the retinal area usually projects. Diplopia occurs when ____________ retinal areas are stimulated.

395. (1) 1
(2) .02

396. Vertical phorias are described in the same manner as the vertical squints, ie, right hypertropia and right hyperphoria; left hypertropia and (1) ____________ (2) ____________ .

544. 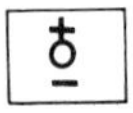

545. If an esotrope shows fusion with the proper testing situation (ie, mirror or prism), it is found that about 70% will fuse and have straight eyes after the proper treatment.

How does the presence of fusion affect the prognosis in a case of esotropia?

692. eccentric fixation

693. If the amblyopic patient is an eccentric fixator, the prognosis for restoration of vision is much poorer than if the patient is a central fixator. How does the type of fixation in the amblyope affect prognosis?

840. tucking

841. In most individuals, the vagus nerve (which slows the heart rate) sends branches to the eye muscles. In those patients, tugging on the eye muscles results in ____________ of the heart rate.

98. (1) 25$^{\triangle}$
(2) esotropia
(3) Krimsky

99. 30$^{\triangle}$ base-in are necessary to center the corneal reflex (reflex is centered in other eye). This patient has an (1) ____________ (type) of (2) ____________ (amount) as measured by the (3) ____________ method.

---

247. noncorresponding

248. Since seeing the same object in two different locations in space is disturbing, the retina-brain system has the ability to shut off the impression of one image. This is known as suppression.

In suppression, the brain-retina system can (1) ____________ the impression from (2) ____________.

---

396. (1) left
(2) hyperphoria

397. With a Maddox rod (grooves vertical) placed over the right eye, the patient looks at a light. The right eye sees a horizontal line of light, and the other eye sees a spot of light.

If a Maddox rod is placed over OD, the (1) ____________ sees a line, and the (2) ____________ sees a spot of light.

545. About 70% will have straight eyes and fusion after the proper treatment (makes prognosis better).

546. Most exotropes will be found to have fusion. Since postoperative fusion is in a large measure dependent on preoperative fusion, exotropes can be predicted to have ______________ postoperatively.

693. Eccentric fixation makes for a poorer prognosis than central fixation.

694. You may recall that abnormal retinal correspondence, which is seen in squint cases, is associated with the development of a pseudo fovea.

In abnormal retinal correspondence, the patient develops a ______________.

841. slowing

842. Cases of eye muscle stimulation resulting in a complete stoppage of the heartbeat have been reported.

Cardiac arrest resulting from tugging on the ______________ has been reported.

99. (1) exotropia
(2) 30^{Δ} (or 15°)
(3) Krimsky

100. The Krimsky method measures squints by ______.

248. (1) shut off (or suppress)
(2) one eye

249. Most patients with squints do not report double vision (diplopia). Although noncorresponding portions of each retina report the same impression to the brain, the brain suppresses one impression.

Most squints do not report diplopia because of the brain mechanism called ______.

397. (1) OD
(2) OS

398. With a Maddox rod placed before an eye of a patient with no vertical deviation, the line would be seen to intersect the light spot.

If the diagrammed pattern is seen with the Maddox rod, is a vertical tropia present?

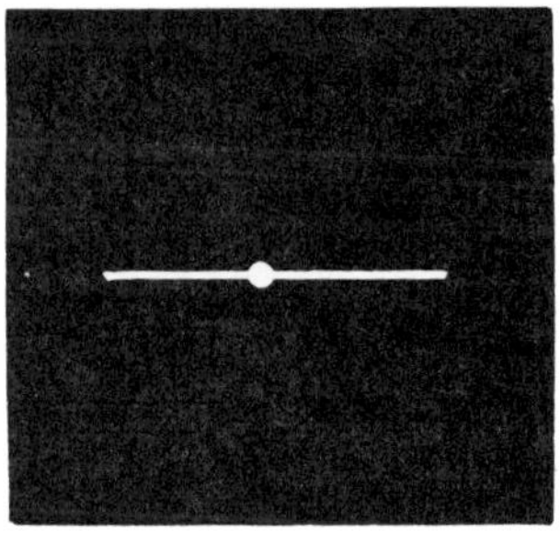

546. fusion

547. It has been pointed out that corresponding retinal areas have the same directional quality in common.

(1) If the nasal retina of the right eye is stimulated by a light, where does the subject think the light is located?

(2) If the temporal retina of the left eye is stimulated by a light, where does the subject think the light is located?

694. pseudo fovea

695. Eccentric fixation is often associated with abnormal retinal correspondence. In both conditions, the patient establishes a pseudo fovea.

What do eccentric fixation and abnormal retinal correspondence have in common?

842. eye muscles

843. Atropine, either preoperatively or at the time of eye muscle manipulation, effectively blocks the vagal-vagal response or heart-slowing reflex. If the pulse slows with eye muscle manipulation, the patient should be immediately given ____________.

100. centering the corneal reflex with prisms (or equivalent words)

101. The measurements of squints are done by means or variations of three basic methods.

(1) Alternate occlusion and neutralization of ocular movements by either prisms or an instrument such as the (a) __________ .

(2) Noting the position of the corneal reflex is called the (b) __________ measurement.

(3) Centering the corneal reflex with prisms is called the (c) __________ measurement.

249. suppression

250. The posterior or occipital portion of the cortex of the brain is known to be involved in the reception and processing of information sent from the retinas. This area of the cortex is called the occipital cortex.

The visual cortex is located in the __________ portion of the cortex.

398. no

399. If the Maddox rod is placed before an eye of a patient with a vertical deviation, the higher image (line or dot) is seen by the eye which deviates down.

When a Maddox rod is before OD and the diagrammed pattern is seen, which eye deviates down?

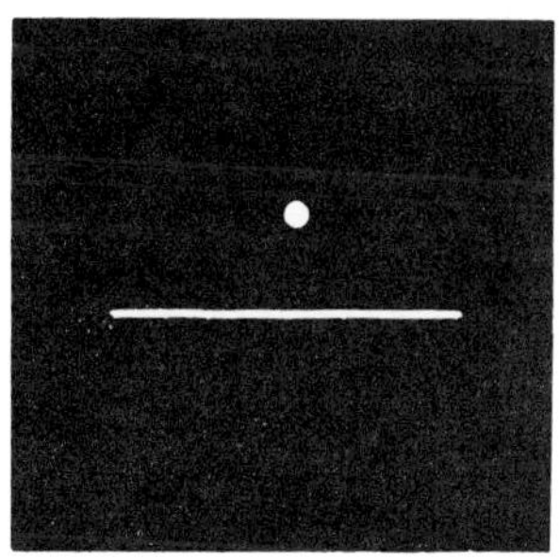

547. (1) to the right
(2) to the right

548. The foveal areas of both eyes are considered corresponding areas when they are stimulated by a target, and the subject has the impression that the target is located straight ahead if his eyes are directed straight ahead.

In this diagram of a normal subject with both eyes converged on the target, where does the subject believe the target is located?

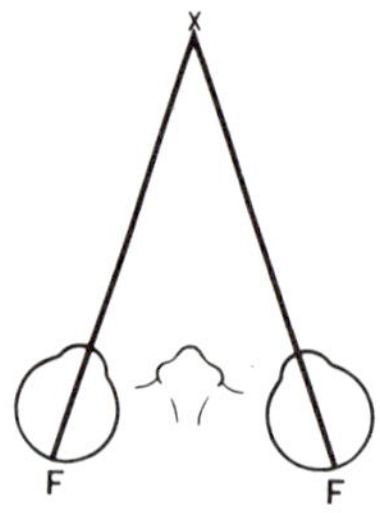

695. pseudo fovea

696. Presence of a pseudo fovea in eccentric fixation implies that the condition is firmly entrenched and makes the prognosis poor.

What effect does the presence of a pseudo fovea have on prognosis?

843. atropine

844. Occasionally, the conjunctiva and lid of an operated eye will start to swell about a week after a muscle operation. This is usually a result of allergy to the catgut suture.

Swelling of an eye one week after eye muscle surgery should make one think of ____________ to the catgut suture.

101. (a) amblyoscope
(b) Hirshberg
(c) Krimsky

102. Neutralizing the movement of the eyes by an appropriate prism when they are alternately covered and uncovered is called the prism-cover test. The strength of the prism which neutralizes movement of the eyes as the eyes are alternately occluded is the same as (1)________. Alternate occlusion accompanied by neutralization of eye movement with prisms is called the (2)________ test.

---

250. occipital

251. Although the exact site for the suppression mechanism in the brain is unknown, it is believed to be in or near the visual (occipital) cortex.

The site for suppression is probably ________.

---

399. OS

400. A convenient method for measuring vertical phoria consists of using a Maddox rod over one eye with the grooves held vertically. If the patient sees the diagrammed pattern with Maddox rod over OD, you know that prism base-________ OD will align the line on the dot. (Remember that a prism displaces an image toward its apex.)

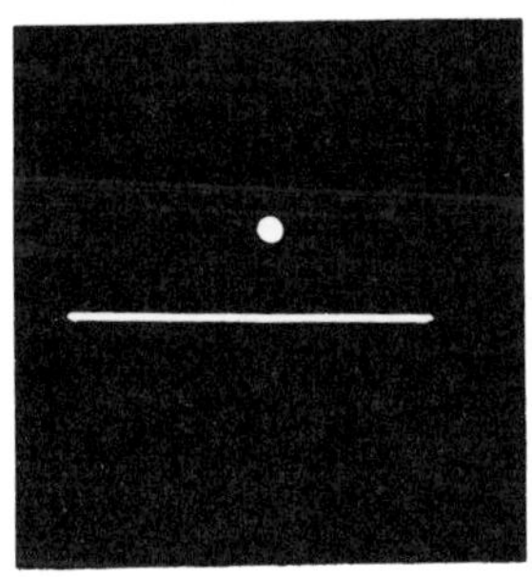

548. straight ahead in the midline

549. If noncorresponding points in each eye are stimulated, and each retinal area retains its specific directional value, diplopia will result. Why is diplopia reported when similar retinal images strike noncorresponding retinal areas?

---

696. makes it poor

697. For treatment purposes, amblyopia must be divided into those patients with central fixation and those patients with eccentric fixation.

For treatment purposes, how is amblyopia divided?

---

844. allergy

845. Anatomic studies show that the anterior segment of the eye (cornea, iris, ciliary body) receives blood from arteries which also supply the four recti.

Arteries supplying the four rectus muscles also supply the ____________ of the eye.

102. (1) the amount of squint
(2) cover test with prisms (prism-cover test)

103. The distance the object of fixation is from the patient will also vary the amount of squint found. Therefore, measurements of squint at both distance (20 feet; *6 meters*) and near (14 inches; *1/3 meter*) are usually made. Measurements of a tropia are taken while the patient is fixating at (1)__________ and while the patient is fixating at (2)__________.

251. in or near the visual cortex

252. As noted before, over 50% of the patients with exotropia have the intermittent variety. When their eyes are straight, their brains fuse images from corresponding parts of their retinas.

In intermittent exotropia, during periods of no squinting, the patients can __________ images from both retinas.

400. down

401. With the Maddox rod over OD, the patient sees as diagrammed. Prism base- (1)__________ OS will align the dot on the line. This patient has a (2)__________ hyperphoria.

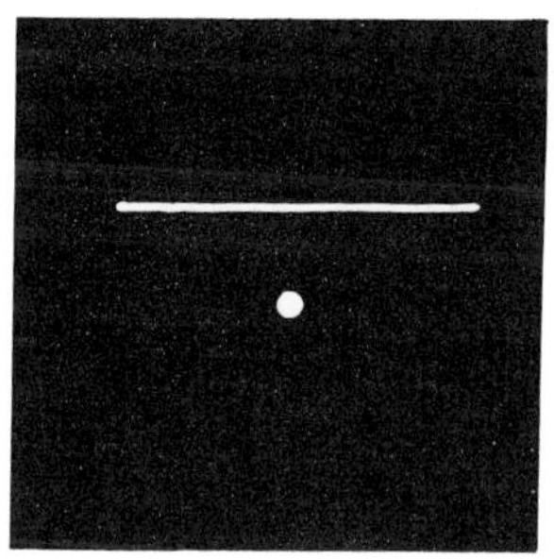

549. When the same image strikes noncorresponding retinal areas, the brain gets the impression that each image comes from a different direction in space.

550. When the fovea of one eye is stimulated by an image, the brain gets the impression that the target is straight ahead if the eye is directed straight ahead. If a point on the nasal retina of the other eye receives the same image, it reports that the target must be temporally located.

Corresponding retinal areas have what in common?

---

697. those with central fixation
those with eccentric fixation

698. For central fixators with amblyopia, treatment consists of constant occlusion of the nonamblyopic eye.

What treatment is used for treating amblyopes with central fixation?

---

845. anterior segment

846. Operations on adult patients which involved surgery to all four rectus muscles have been known to interfere with the blood supply to the anterior segment, causing permanent damage.

It is unwise to operate on all ____________ rectus muscles at one time.

103. (1) distance (20 feet; 6 meters) } either
(2) near (14 inches; ⅓ meter) } order

104. XT is an abbreviation for exotropia as measured while the patient fixates at distance (6 meters), and XT′ is an abbreviation for exotropia measured while the patient fixates at near (1/3 meter). Likewise, ET indicates esotropia measured while the patient fixates at (1) ____________, and ET′ means the esotropia was measured with the patient fixating at (2) ____________.

252. fuse

253. If you were to examine an intermittent exotrope when he was squinting, you might be able to get him to see double. In truth, diplopia may be elicited in almost 50% of all exotropes.

Under the proper testing situation, about how many out of a group of 100 exotropes would report diplopia?

401. (1) down
(2) left

402. Vertical fusional reserves can be measured at near or at distance and will usually be about the same. A prism, base-up, before either eye, is increased with the rotatory prism until the patient reports diplopia. The prism base-up is then reduced until single vision is reported. The same procedure is repeated with a prism base-down over the same eye. The above describes how to measure ____________.

550. When stimulated, they report that the stimulus comes from the same location in space.

551. Animals appear to be born with a fixed relationship between corresponding retinal areas; however, it is questionable that humans have such a fixed relationship at birth, since some patients with squints seem to be able to develop a correspondence between what would normally be noncorresponding areas.

(1) Is normal retinal correspondence present at birth in animals? (2) In humans?

---

698. constant occlusion of the nonamblyopic eye

699. Patching is a term used to denote occlusion of an eye. The patch is usually made of an adhesive to keep it securely in place. The patient in the photo has the right eye occluded or ______________.

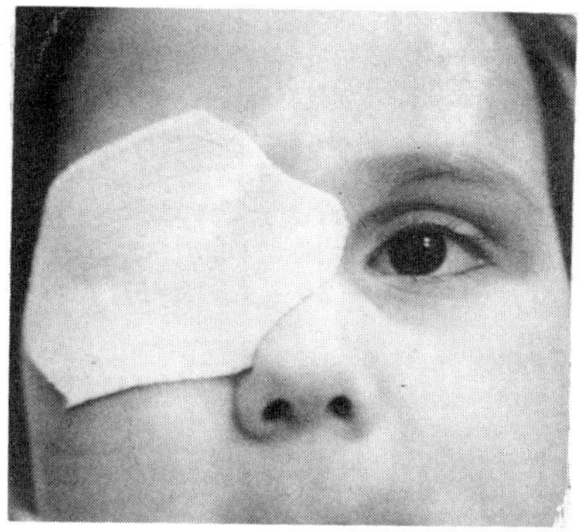

---

846. four

847. Strong controversy rages over the surgical treatment of significant amounts of **A** or **V** syndrome. Operations involving every one of the eye muscles have been suggested at one time or another.

Specific types of surgical management for **A** and **V** syndromes (are/are not) universally accepted.

104. (1) distance (or 6 M)
(2) near (or 1/3 M)

105. A measurement of 15△ XT indicates there is 15△ (1) ____________ (type squint), with the patient fixating at (2) ____________.

A measurement of 25△ ET′ indicates there is 25△ (3) ____________ (type squint), when the patient fixates at (4) ____________.

253. 50

254. The facts indicate that in most cases of exotropia, the mechanism of suppression is not fully or constantly used.

Since exotropes can fuse when their eyes are straight and often see double when one eye turns out, the mechanism of ____________ is not in full or constant use.

402. vertical fusional reserves

403. Vertical fusional reserves are not affected by accommodation, so the distance and near vertical fusional reserves would be expected to be ____________.

551. (1) yes
(2) questionable (probably not)

552. In a case of esotropia, if a nasal retinal area in the turned eye develops an abnormal correspondence with the fovea of the fixing eye, then stimulating either of these areas will give the impression of the target being straight ahead. In the diagram, the point *M* in the OS has developed an abnormal correspondence with the fovea in OD. If *M* is stimulated by the target *X*, where will the subject think *X* is located?

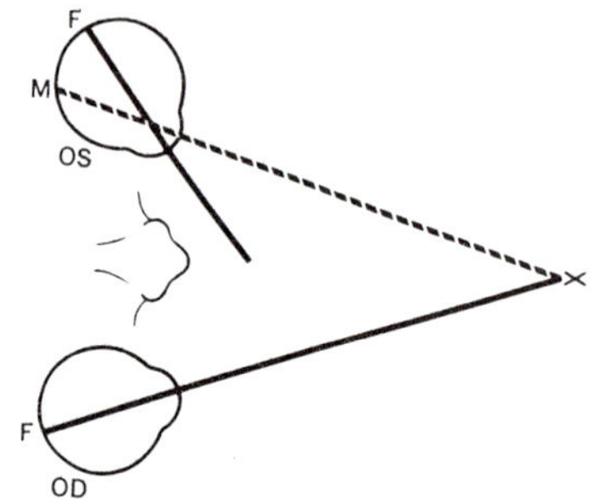

699. patched

700. The concept behind the patching treatment is to force the amblyopic eye to develop normal visual activity by constant work.

By patching the good eye, the amblyopic eye is forced to ____________.

847. are not

848. Most experts feel that if abnormal overaction of any of the vertical acting muscles can be demonstrated in a case of **A** or **V** syndrome, these muscles should be recessed.

In a case of a V-eso syndrome with demonstrated overaction of both inferior obliques, surgery would involve correction of the ET plus (1) ____________ of both (2) ____________ .

105. (1) exotropia (3) esotropia
(2) distance (or 6 M) (4) near (or 1/3 M)

106. This is a photo of a 40△ ET, which means the esotropia was measured while the patient fixated on ____________ .

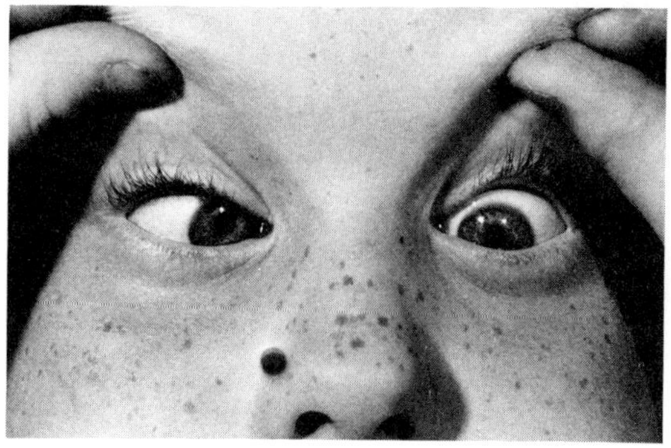

254. suppression

255. Many exotropes complain that their eyes bother them. If they often see double to a slight or great degree, this would tend to be a very frustrating way of looking at the world. Not seeing properly naturally leads to some sort of eye complaint.

Eye complaints from many exotropes may stem from their ____________.

403. the same (or similar)

404. Vertical fusional reserves are usually recorded as BU OD 6/4. This means that 6△ base-up OD caused diplopia, and that 4△ base-up OD returned single vision.

What would a vertical fusion reading of BU OD 7/3 mean?

552. straight ahead

553. In the case of normal retinal correspondence in a squinting patient, stimulation of the foveal area of the deviated eye is suppressed.

Why does stimulation of the fovea of the deviating eye not cause confusion in a patient who has normal retinal correspondence?

---

700. work constantly (and hopefully develop normal visual activity)

701. The patch should be worn 24 hours a day. For effective patching, what part of the day must the child wear a patch?

---

848. (1) recession (disinsertion, or weakening)
(2) inferior obliques

849. Good results are often obtained in A-exo deviations by weakening the overacting superior obliques. Surgical management includes correction of the exotropia superior gaze position and ____________ of both superior obliques.

106. an object at infinity (or distance of 6 M)

107.

PART II
FUSION AND PHORIAS

(Advance to next frame.)

255. diplopia

256. Commonly, if a patient with a squint easily suppresses one retinal image, he does not complain of his eyes feeling tired or painful.

Why don't patients with squints who easily suppress one image complain of eye strain?

404. 7△ BU caused diplopia.
3△ BU returned single vision.

405. Vertical fusional reserves are usually 3-6△ in amount, with base-down measurements the same as base-up if no phoria is present. If the vertical fusional reserve measures 5△ base-up OD for diplopia, and recovery is reported at 3△ base-up, the reserves base-down OD should measure (1) ____________ △ base-down for diplopia and (2) ____________ △ base-down for recovery.

553. Its impression is suppressed.

554. As noted before, because of the natural construction of the retina and brain, the fovea is the most sensitive part of the retina for picking up small details.

(1) If a new area on a retina develops a correspondence with the fovea of the other eye, does it develop the sensitivity of the fovea?

(2) Why?

---

701. 24 hours (or equivalent words)

702. Patching is most effective when the patch is applied directly on the skin over the eye. A patch over a lens is less effective since the patient can look over or around the occluder. When possible, occlusion should be ____________ .

---

849. recessions (or tenotomies)

850. Many experts feel that simply correcting a horizontal squint with surgery will correct an **A** or **V** pattern of less than 15△.

Would you expect a recession-resection operation on an **A**-eso to correct the **A** component of 35△?

(*Advance to next frame.*)

108. A single image is perceived if each eye is fixating on an object with the fovea, and the eyes have the usual retinal correspondence. This ability to see an object as one (although both retinas are used simultaneously) is called fusion. The perception of two retinal images (one in each eye) as a single image is called ___________.

256. There is no bothersome diplopia (or equivalent words).

257. Although it may sound strange, over 50% of exotropes can be made to fuse retinal images while they are squinting. To accomplish this, we must get similar images onto corresponding retinal areas of both eyes.

If (1) ___________ retinal areas are stimulated with (2) ___________, over 50% of squinting exotropes can fuse.

405. (1) 5
(2) 3

406. If the vertical phoria is ortho, the vertical fusional reserves are expected to be equal; conversely, if the base-up OD fusional reserves equalled the base-down OD fusional reserves, you would expect the vertical phoria to be ___________.

554. (1) no
(2) The inherent anatomy of the fovea and its brain connections are different (or similar wording).

555. Although a new point on a retina takes up correspondence with the fovea of the other eye, its vision never approaches that of the fovea.

Abnormally corresponding retinal areas stimulated by the same target have the same spatial direction, but the vision of the retinal area abnormally corresponding to the fovea of the other eye is

____________.

---

702. directly on the skin over the eye

703. As long as improvement in vision continues, constant patching is continued. A plateau of no further improvement over two months typically indicates maximal visual acuity. When do you stop patching?

---

850. no

851. If the patient had an A-eso of about 20△, the surgeon might do bimedial recessions and at the same time move the insertions of the medial recti up.

In an A-eso the ET is greater in the elevated position; therefore, moving the medial recti up must ____________ their action when the eye looks up.

108. fusion

109. Only if both retinal images are fused into a single image can the third dimension be perceived. In most instances the two retinal images are quite similar, differing only in the slight angle of viewing caused by the separation of the two eyes. These slight differences in the two retinal images give clues as to depth (depth perception).

A prerequisite for depth perception is (1) __________ of the slightly different images. These differences are caused by (2) __________ .

---

257. (1) corresponding
(2) similar images

258. Suppose that we place a 40 diopter prism base-in before an eye which has turned out 40 prism diopters and flash a target before the patient. An image of that target will fall on corresponding retinal areas. In the diagram, an appropriate prism has allowed the image of *X* to be on __________ retinal areas.

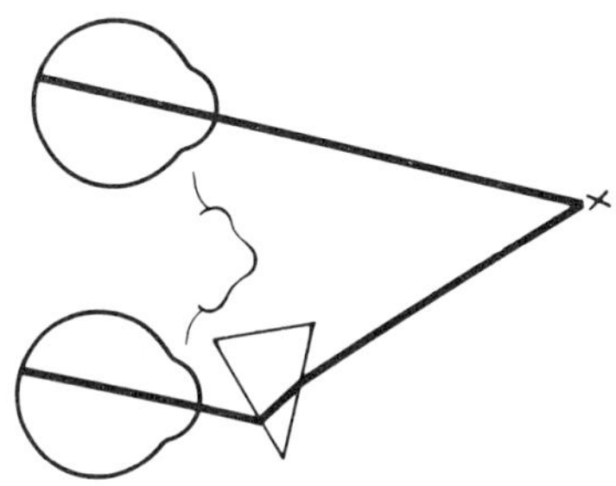

---

406. zero (or ortho)

407. If the base-up OS fusional reserves equalled the base-down OS fusional reserves, you would expect the vertical phoria to be __________ .

555. poorer

556. An amblyoscope is a device in which each eye can only see its target and not the target of the other eye. This is accomplished by having each eye look at a target at the end of a tube.

In the simple illustration, how can the target in the amblyoscope be placed along the visual axis of the deviating eye?

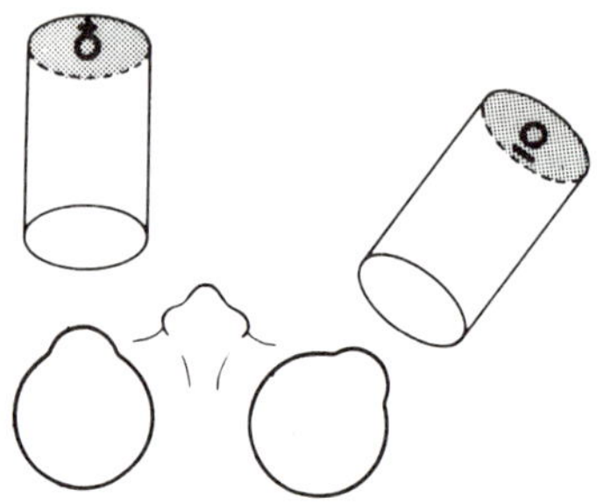

703. after 2 months of no further improvement

704. Success of the patching treatment in amblyopia will depend upon the age of the child. Best results are obtained in children under 12.

Success in patching central fixators is related to the ____________ of the patient.

851. weaken

852. When no squint is present in the straight ahead position, but an incapacitating squint (eso or exo) exists in the depressed reading position, simply moving the appropriate recti (1) ____________ or (2) ____________ may produce a cure.

109. (1) fusion
(2) separation of the two eyes giving different views (or similar wording)

110. A newborn child seems to have the ability to utilize the two eyes together although not in a precise manner. The testing of fusion in the newborn is difficult, but some evidence suggests that a surprisingly good degree of depth perception is often present. By three months of age, most children have well coordinated eye movements and reasonably good fusion.

If a satisfactory test for depth perception existed you (would/would not) expect a three-month-old child to pass the test.

---

258. corresponding

259. We can get a target to fall on corresponding visual axes by using a mirror. By rotating a mirror the proper amount, it will reflect light from the target to the fovea of the squinting eye. By calibrating a rotating mirror device, one could measure the ____________ of a squint when the patient reported fusion of a target.

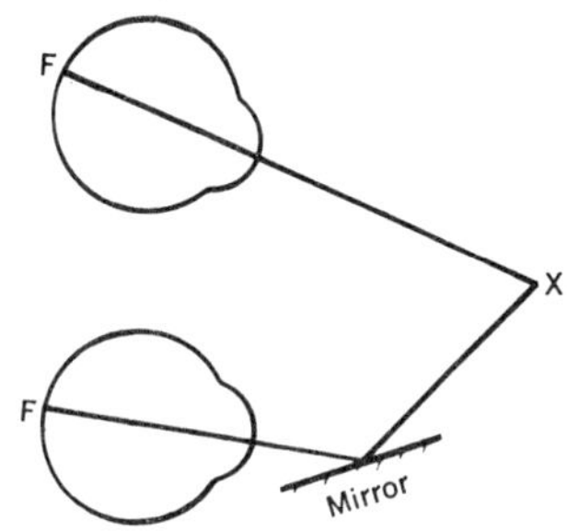

---

407. zero (or ortho)

408. If a patient exhibits a vertical phoria, then the patient's vertical fusional reserves are expected to be altered proportionally. A patient who has a $1^{\triangle}$ right hyperphoria and had a base-up OD fusional reserve of 4/2 would be expected to have a base-down fusional reserve of 5/3. If a patient has a left hyperphoria, the OS (base-up/base-down) fusional reserves would be expected to be greater.

556. by moving the tube

557. In a case of squint with fusion, if each tube of the amblyoscope is lined up along the visual axis of each eye, the patient will be able to fuse.

If the esotrope in the illustration has fusion, what letter will he report if the tubes are lined up along his visual axis? (*L*/*F*/*E*)

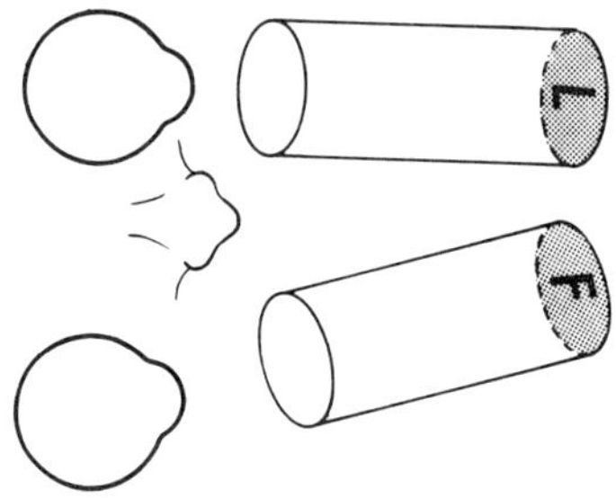

704. age

705. Generally, in patients under 12, patching should improve vision considerably in the amblyopic eye in about $\frac{3}{4}$ of the cases.

In a group of 100 amblyopic patients under 12 who receive patching treatment, how many should show an improvement?

852. (1) up } either
(2) down } order

853. In the case of an **A**-eso condition where the squint is greater in the elevated position, recess the medial recti and move them ______________ .

110. would

111. The perception of the third dimension allows us to appreciate relative depth. The sense of the third dimension is called ____________ .

259. angle

260. One could also measure the angle of a squint by using a rotating mirror and the cover test.

In a case of squint, if the rotating mirror were directing rays from the target to the fovea of the squinting eye and the fixating eye were covered, the deviating eye would ____________ .

408. base-down

409. A patient has a 2△ right hyperphoria. The base-up OD fusional reserves are 4/2. The base-down OD fusional reserves would be expected to be (less/greater) than 4/2.

557. E

558. In a case of squint without fusion, if the tubes are lined up along the patient's visual axes, he will maintain suppression of the squinting eye.

If the exotrope in the diagram does not have fusion, what will he see? (y/ʌ/X) (OD is the deviating eye)

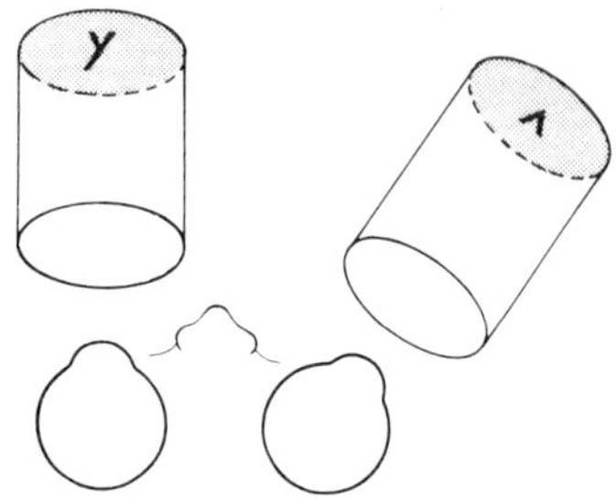

705. about 75

706. It must be appreciated that visual improvement is relative. A patient who goes from 20/200 to 20/40 is just as much a success as one who goes from 20/40 to 20/20. Do all therapeutic successes in amblyopic patients attain 20/20 vision?

853. up

854. In a case of A-eso, if the surgeon wants to work with the lateral recti, he would resect them and move the insertions ____________, thereby making the lateral recti stronger in upward gaze.

111. depth perception (or stereopsis)

112. Grade I fusion means that the patient has simultaneous macular perception. If the patient sees figure *A* (Grade I target) with OD and sees figure *B* (Grade I target) with OS, sketch what he will see with Grade I fusion.

A 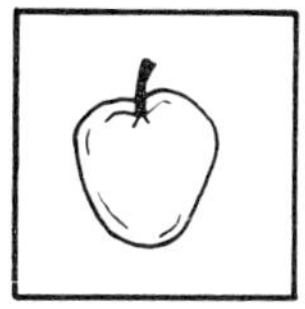

B 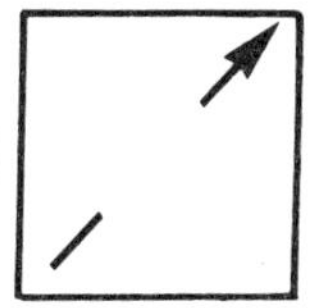

260. not move

261. It appears that if we trace most cases of exotropia, we see that they were born with straight eyes. During their early years one eye turns out on occasion. The condition progresses so that one eye (at any one time) turns out more frequently.

As exotropia develops, the periods of straight eyes (1) ____________ , and the periods of exotropia (2) ____________ .

409. greater

410. Since vertical fusional reserves are low (compared to the size of horizontal fusional reserves), you would expect a small vertical phoria (to be/ not to be) symptomatic.

558. Y

559. In a squint with abnormal retinal correspondence (ARC), a nonfoveal area of one eye has developed a sense of direction similar to that of the fixing eye. The patient in the illustration has an esotropia. He reports seeing B with the tubes straight. What condition does he have?

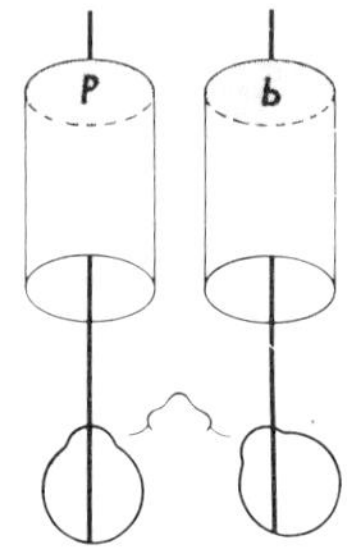

706. no

707. Although adult patients with amblyopia have a poor prognosis, it should be mentioned that patients as old as 60 have achieved substantial improvement. Although seldom indicated, can a patient over 12 with amblyopia hope for improvement in vision with treatment?

854. down

855. The rule to follow in moving horizontal muscles up and down in the **V** and **A** patterns is to move the muscle in the direction you wish to weaken it. To weaken a medial rectus on downward gaze you would move the medial rectus ___________.

112. 

113. If a patient can fuse Grade I targets with a 10^{Δ} prism, base-in (BI), in front of one eye, and can also fuse the same targets with a 10^{Δ} prism, base-out (BO), we would say he has 10^{Δ} BI and 10^{Δ} BO fusional reserve. Grade I fusion with fusional reserve equals Grade II fusion.

He has at least Grade ____________ fusion.

---

261. (1) decrease
(2) increase

262. An intermittent exotrope will have straight eyes most of the time. Generally, the eye will turn out when the child is tired or daydreaming. Often he can straighten his eyes on command.

When does an intermittent exotrope usually squint?

---

410. to be

411. The symptoms of a vertical phoria may range from feelings of eye strain to intermittent diplopia. If the vertical fusional reserves are sufficient, the patient (will/will not) complain of vertical diplopia.

559. ARC

560. When a patient with ARC and a squint is placed in the amblyoscope and he reports fusion when the tubes are both straight, the condition is called harmonious ARC.

A patient reports fusion when the tube before the deviating eye is straight. The patient has ____________ ARC.

707. yes

708. Patching the good eye will usually have no deleterious effects on that eye. But occasional cases have been recorded where the good eye became amblyopic. For that reason, the patched eye must be checked frequently to ascertain that its vision is ____________.

855. down

856. In the case of a **V**-eso with the ET being greater in the depressed position, the surgeon would recess the medial recti and move their insertions ____________.

113. II

114. Grade I fusion means only that the patient can perceive two dissimilar retinal images as a single image without fusional reserve or depth perception. If the right eye sees figure *A*, and the left eye sees figure *B*, then a patient with Grade I fusion would see these Grade I targets as ________________.
(sketch)

A
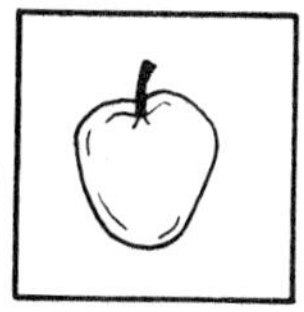

B
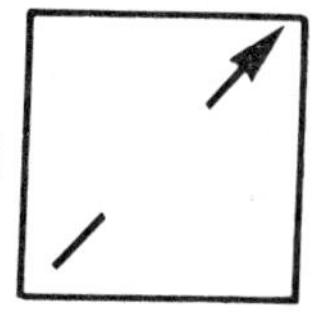

262. during periods of fatigue or daydreaming

263. As exotropia develops, it usually follows one of two paths. Either the patient squints first when looking into the distance, or he squints first when looking at near objects.

What are the two common forms that a developing exotropia may take?

411. will not

412. Since small vertical phorias may be symptomatic, any artificially induced vertical phoria may be symptomatic. Thus, poorly fitted glasses may produce a vertical prismatic effect which is different for the two eyes. Such glasses may produce a ________________ phoria and symptoms.

560. harmonious

561. In the majority of cases of known congenital vertical muscle palsy, fusion was maintained by a compensatory head turn, and no horizontal squint developed.

In a majority of patients with a congenital palsy of a vertically acting muscle, is a horizontal squint present?

708. not decreasing (or equivalent words)

709. The worsening of vision of the patched good eye is called occlusion amblyopia. Occlusion amblyopia can be minimized by checking the vision of both eyes at intervals corresponding to one week for every year of age of the patient. Occlusion amblyopia should be considered in every patched eye. Amblyopia treatment consists of a vision check every ____________ weeks when treating a three-year-old child.

856. down

857. In the case of an A-exo with the XT greater in the down position, the surgeon might recess the lateral recti and move the insertions ____________. (Remember the rule: **Move the muscle in the direction you wish to weaken it.**)

114. 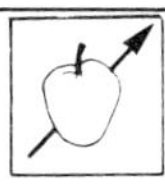

115. The ability to fuse two retinal images (one in each eye) into one and to perceive depth is regarded as Grade III fusion. A lesser amount of fusion (Grade II) consists of perceiving one image from the two retinal images with fusional reserve. In Grade II fusion, the eyes can be made to diverge or converge and still utilize both foveal images and perceive one, but without depth perception.

Grade III fusion means the patient has ____________ .

263. (1) start as exotropia when looking far away
(2) start as exotropia when looking at near objects
} either order

264. The type of exotropia that starts when looking at distant objects is called **exotropia with divergence excess.** The patient is able to converge his eyes to a near object, but turns an eye out too much when looking far away.

In divergence excess, the patient is usually exotropic at ____________ .

412. vertical (or hyper)

413. Since glasses may produce a significant vertical phoria, it is well to check the vertical phoria with the patient first wearing his own glasses and then wearing his prescription in a trial frame.

If vertical phoria is suspected, always check for vertical phoria with the patient wearing ____________ first.

561. no

562. To complicate the picture, in the amblyoscope, some cases of ARC neither align the tubes straight ahead nor do they align the tubes with the visual axes of both eyes, but fall somewhere in between. This condition is called **unharmonious ARC.**

In unharmonious ARC, how is a tube lined up before the deviating eye?

709. three

710. In treating an amblyope with eccentric fixation, the first task is to convert the fixation into a central type.

What is the first step in treating amblyopia with eccentric fixation?

857. down

858. The surgical treatment of vertical squints is similar to that for horizontal squints. Recessions or resections are employed as needed, depending on the muscle which needs to be strengthened. The operation to strengthen an inferior rectus would be a __________ of that muscle.

115. depth perception (or stereopsis)

116. Instruments used to view separate fusion targets with each eye and to move them are called haploscopes or diploscopes.

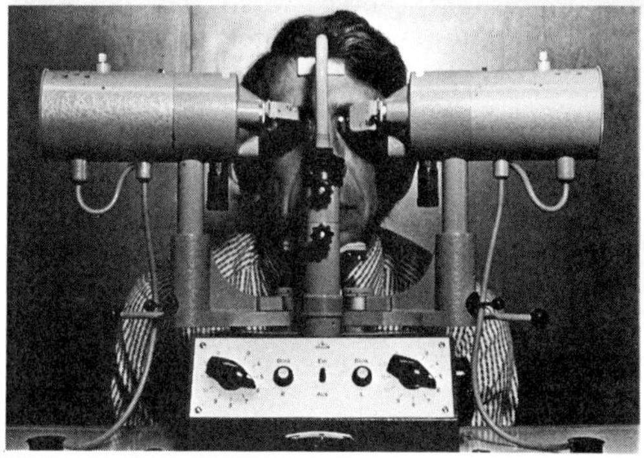

The diploscope to present targets and measure fusional amplitude shown in frame 62 was an amblyoscope. The diploscope shown here is a synoptophore. Both the amblyoscope and the synoptophore are called ____________ .

264. distance viewing

265. The patient who starts out by being exotropic only when looking at close objects is considered to be of the **convergence insufficiency** type.

In convergence insufficiency, the exotropia is noted during ____________ .

413. his usual glasses (or equivalent wording)

414.

PART VI
COMITANT VS. NONCOMITANT SQUINTS

(Advance to next frame.)

562. at some point other than straight ahead and the direction of the patient's visual axis

563. As we have noted, when the fixing eye is covered, the deviating eye directs its fovea toward the object of regard. In doing so, suppression of the foveal impression is either partially or fully stopped, for suppression is not necessary if the eye is covered.

A squint with both eyes open usually suppresses the (1)____________ area of the (2)____________ eye. (3) If the fixing eye is covered, does suppression take place in either eye?

---

710. convert fixation to central type

711. If the patient with eccentric fixation is under five, patching the amblyopic eye for a few weeks and then patching the good eye while uncovering the amblyopic eye may restore normal fixation.

In a patient under five with eccentric fixation, which eye would you patch first?

---

858. resection

859. The operation to weaken an inferior rectus muscle would be a ____________ of that muscle.

116. diploscopes (or haploscopes or stereoscopes)

117. If a person's two eyes cannot bring images together into a single image, he may have diplopia (double vision). Diplopia is frequently produced as a means of testing certain parameters of binocular vision. If we place more prism diopters in front of a patient than he has fusional reserve, he may report ______ .

265. near viewing

266. In time, the patient who has an exotropia at near often develops one for distance viewing and the patient with an exotropia at distance develops one for near viewing.

In the course of development, most convergence insufficiencies and divergence excess cases develop squints ______ .

414. (*Advance to next frame.*)

415. If the eyes deviate the same amount, irrespective of the direction of gaze, the squint is said to be comitant. A squint which is 12△ ET straight ahead, up, down, left, and right is said to be a 12△ ______ esotropia.

563. (1) foveal
(2) deviating (or squinting)
(3) no

. . . .

564. A patient with a squint and ARC can also pick up fixation with the fovea of the deviating eye when the other eye is covered.

Can you tell whether a patient has ARC from doing a cover test?

---

711. amblyopic eye

. . . .

712. The concept behind patching the amblyopic eye in eccentric fixation is to prevent the patient from continuing the bad pattern of eccentric fixation so that he can subsequently develop a normal fixation pattern. When the patch is removed, it is hoped that the patient again fixates in the normal central fashion.

What is to be gained by patching the amblyopic eye?

---

859. recession

. . . .

860. Recession of an inferior rectus muscle must be conservative. If an excessive recession is performed, the lower lid tends to droop down. Four mm is considered by some to be the maximum safe recession of an inferior rectus. A recession of an inferior rectus in excess of __________ mm is seldom necessary. If more is needed, then special dissection is required.

117. diplopia

118. Fusion can be interrupted by presenting a totally different target to each eye. When fusion is interrupted the eyes are said to be dissociated. The absence of fusion implies ____________ of the eyes.

266. for both near and distance viewing

267. There is a group of exophoric patients who never squint. They show a controlled tendency to turn an eye out during distance or near viewing. The terms convergence insufficiency and divergence excess are also applied to them, however, without the use of the term exotropia.

A nonsquinting exophoric patient can have (1) ____________ excess or (2) ____________ insufficiency.

415. comitant

416. A squint which varies as the patient changes his direction of gaze is said to be incomitant or noncomitant. If a patient has $10^{\triangle}$ ET looking straight ahead, but $15^{\triangle}$ XT looking up, he is said to have a(n) ____________ squint.

564. no

565. The fovea of the deviating eye in ARC takes on a new sense of direction, just as the area corresponding to the fovea of the fixing eye takes on a straight ahead sensitivity. The area of the deviating eye which corresponds to the fovea of the straight eye is called the pseudo fovea.

In a patient with ARC, which area of the retina in the turned eye has a straight ahead sensation?

---

712. not to allow the patient to continue the eccentric fixation pattern (or equivalent words)

713. Even if the central fixation is not established, the usual treatment of patching the good eye is started after five weeks of patching the amblyopic eye.

When do you patch the good eye in treating amblyopia?

---

860. 4

861. Which eye should be attacked surgically for a hypotropia? The eye which is not fixing is the rule. If the patient has a right hypertropia and fixes with OD you would advise surgery on ____________.

118. dissociation

119. The tendency to see singly is great; thus, to examine the properties of binocular vision some method for dissociation is necessary. One method of dissociation is to present dissimilar targets to the eyes, such as having one eye see a line, the other a dot of light. The eyes will be dissociated because the line and dot are __________ targets.

267. (1) divergence
(2) convergence

268. There are many different ways that patients' eyes may turn out. One patient's eye may turn out when looking at a far-off target, only on occasion or always; another's may turn out when doing a near task, intermittently or constantly; another's eye may intermittently or constantly turn out for all types of seeing; or another's may show a tendency to follow one of these patterns, but never actually turn out. Any one patient will exhibit a set pattern which must be checked at (near/distance/near and distance) viewing.

416. incomitant (or noncomitant)

417. A rather common type of incomitant squint is produced by overaction of the inferior obliques. When such a patient looks to his right, the left eye goes up; when he looks to his left, the right eye goes up. This is a(n) (1) __________ squint caused by overaction of the (2) __________ muscles.

565. pseudo fovea (the area now abnormally corresponding to the fovea of the fixing eye)

566. If a target is placed along the visual axis of each eye in a patient with ARC, the two targets will not be superimposed.

If a vertical line | is presented to the fovea of the fixing eye and a horizontal line —— is presented to the fovea of the deviating eye, what will the ARC patient report?

---

713. after 5 weeks of patching the amblyopic eye

714. If central fixation cannot be established by the patching technique, then the red filter technique is used. The good eye is patched and a red filter placed over the amblyopic eye. In the red filter technique, the (1) ____________ eye is patched and the red filter is over the (2) ____________ eye.

---

861. OS

862. A patient with a left hypotropia who prefers OD for fixation would be advised to have surgery on ____________.

119. dissimilar (or different)

120. A horizontal deviation of dissociated eyes can be measured with the appropriate base-in or base-out prism. When the patient sees a dot with one eye and a vertical line with the other, a prism equal to his ocular deviation will align the dot on the ______________.

268. near and distance

269. The many forms of exotropia suggest that one form may lead into another, the last stage being constant exotropia at near and distance. It also appears that a case may become arrested at any stage.

If a child is seen with exotropia for distance viewing only, what can you tell the mother about the future development of the case?

417. (1) incomitant (or noncomitant)
(2) inferior oblique

418. A squint which is constant in all fields of gaze is said to be (1) ______________, while the squint that varies as the patient directs his gaze into different fields is said to be (2) ______________.

566. |—— or ——|

567. When you look up at the sun and then look at a light wall, you often get the impression of a black ball on the wall. The black spot is called the **after-image** of the bright stimulus and corresponds to the shape of the stimulus.

If you looked at a bright vertical light for a few seconds and then looked away, what would you see?

---

714. (1) good
(2) amblyopic

715. The theory for success of the red filter technique is that only the cones respond to red light, hence the eye will use the fovea. When the fixation becomes central the red filter is removed, but the patching of the ____________ eye is continued until the maximal visual improvement is obtained. While theoretically sound, this technique seldom works any better than simple 24-hour per day patching.

---

862. OS

863. A paretic squint is attacked by strengthening the paretic muscle, weakening its antagonist, or by appropriate strengthening or weakening of the yoke muscle.

The surgery for a paretic right superior oblique would be a recession of the left ____________ if the patient preferred to fixate with OD. (Recall that yoke muscles move the eyes in the same direction; for example, down and left.)

120. line (vertical line)

121. If a light is viewed through a glass rod, a streak of light is seen perpendicular to the length of the rod. The reason for this is that the rod is a high-powered cylindrical lens which focuses one linear image parallel to the rod and just behind it (about 10 mm or less from the eye). The eye would require 1000/10 or at least 100 diopters of power to focus it. The other meridian not affected by the lens would be seen as a streak. The image of light seen through a rod is a streak __________ to the rod.

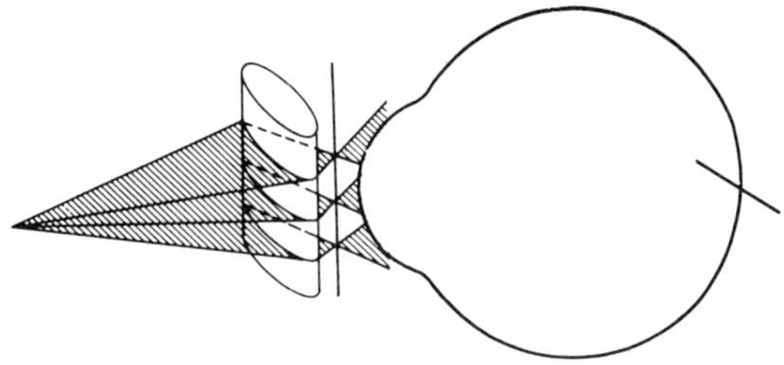

269. Progress may stop at this stage, or the case may go on to a constant exotropia at distance and at near.

270. An adult with convergence insufficiency and no exotropia probably has an arrested case which will not progress. Generally, there is little progress of the condition after the teens.

At what age can you predict with some assurance that convergence insufficiency will not develop into a squint?

418. (1) comitant
(2) incomitant (or noncomitant)

419. The division between comitant vs. incomitant squints depends on variations in the squint in various fields, but not upon the distance to the target. An esotrope of 20△ at distance and 10△ at near may be either comitant or incomitant depending on variations of the squint in __________ .

567. a black vertical line

568. In the after-image test, the turned eye is covered while the other eye fixates on a bright vertical light. Next, the fixating eye is covered and the deviating eye turns to fixate on a horizontal light.

(1) In a patient with normal correspondence, what after-image pattern will be reported?

(2) In a patient with abnormal retinal correspondence, what after-image pattern will be reported?

---

715. good

716. If central fixation cannot be established by a patching technique, then a type of treatment called **pleoptics** is used.

When is pleoptics used in treating eccentric fixation?

---

863. inferior rectus

864. A paretic right superior oblique would be attacked by a disinsertion, recession, or myotomy of the __________ muscle if the patient preferred to fixate with OS.

(Operate on the antagonist of the paretic eye muscle if the nonparetic eye fixates, on the yoke muscle of the paretic muscle if the paretic eye fixates.)

121. perpendicular

122. The Maddox rod is a series of rods or grooves and functions just as a single rod, giving a linear image of a spot of light. The image is ______________ to the axis of the rods.

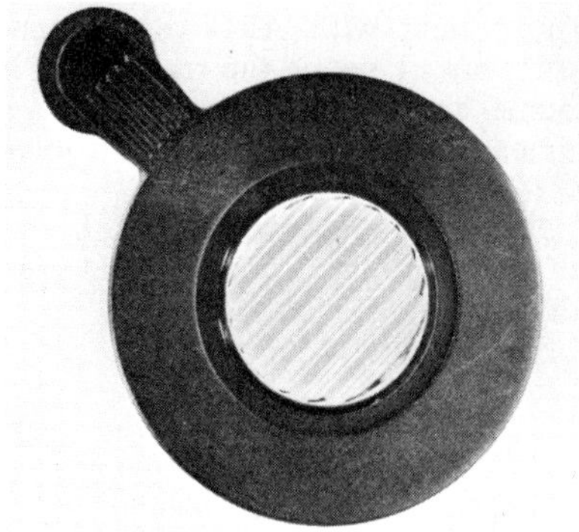

270. after the teens

271. The fovea is the most sensitive viewing area of the retina. The fovea can send more detailed information to the brain about an image than any other part of the retina.

What is meant by saying that the fovea is the most sensitive part of the retina?

419. different fields of gaze

420. The majority of squints are comitant; only about 1% of the squints are incomitant (excluding **A** and **V** squints, which will be considered later). About 99% of all squints are ______________ in various fields of gaze.

568. (1) 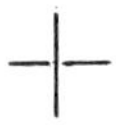 (2) 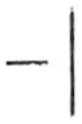 or 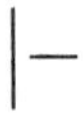

569. The patient with ARC has an unusual yet successful way of seeing the real world. He never sees double and he may have a crude sense of three-dimensionality in a cueless environment.

Could a squint patient with ARC have a crude sense of depth in an environment (1) with cues, (2) without cues?

---

716. if patients cannot restore normal fixation by patching techniques

717. The term *pleoptics* is derived from the Greek and means "full sight." Pleoptics attempts to re-establish foveal fixation.

What is the goal of pleoptics?

---

864. right inferior oblique

865. A paretic right superior oblique could be treated surgically most adequately with a (1)____________ of the (2)____________ muscle if the patient fixated with OD.

122. perpendicular

123. The Maddox rod serves well as a means of dissociating the eyes. If you place a Maddox rod (frequently tinted red) in front of the right eye (with the rods horizontal), while having the patient view a small light at a distance, the image on the retinas will be (*see diagram*):

If the patient has Grade I fusion, he will see both (1) ________ and (2) ________ .

271. It can send more detailed information to the brain about an image than any other part of the retina.

272. If, while you are driving and looking straight ahead, a child should step off the sidewalk, your eyes automatically will turn to the child so that his image will fall on the fovea of each retina.

The fixation reflex automatically turns the eyes so that any new stimulus is focused on the ________ of the retina.

420. the same (or comitant)

421. If any one extraocular muscle is paralyzed, the patient will have a squint which will become worse as he looks in the field of action of the palsied muscle. This will be a(n) ________ squint.

569. (1) yes
(2) probably yes

570. Most squints eventually develop some adaptive way of using both eyes. Even those that appear to suppress the vision in the deviated eye must, in some fashion, use the deviated eye because they notice a difference when that eye is patched.

Is it possible that peripheral retinal areas in a turned eye operate while the central areas are suppressed?

---

717. to reestablish foveal fixation

718. A part of the pleoptic treatment consists of teaching the patient that the true fovea represents a spatial direction straight ahead when the eye is pointed straight ahead. The patient who learns that the true fovea represents a direction straight ahead will direct the fovea to the object of fixation and will have ____________ fixation.

---

865. (1) recession
(2) left inferior rectus

866. **Orthoptics** is a branch of ophthalmology which deals with the establishment of binocular vision nonsurgically. The word is derived from the Greek meaning "straight eye."

Eye exercises and other ____________ surgical techniques are used in orthoptics.

123. (1) the light } either
(2) the red streak } order

124. With the Maddox rod in front of the right eye, the patient's eyes are dissociated. If he has at least Grade I fusion and his visual axes remain aligned with the target, he will see which image? (*A/B/C*)

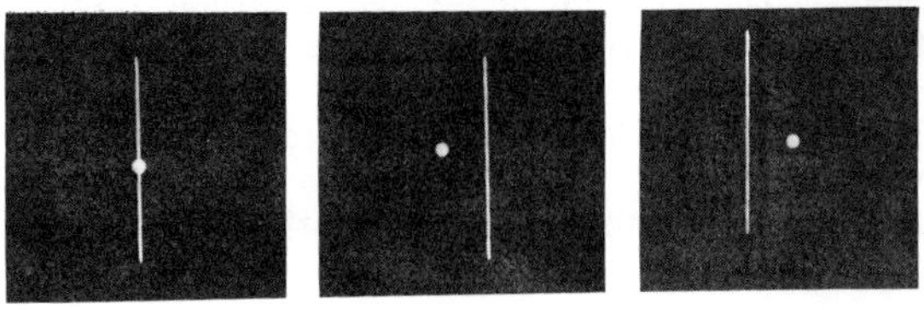

A B C

---

272. fovea

273. The fixation reflex is responsible for bringing an image onto the fovea of each eye and holding it there.

If an object is flashed off to the right, does just the right eye or do both eyes make an attempt to get the image on the fovea or foveas?

---

421. incomitant (or noncomitant or paralytic)

422. Any squint resulting from a paralyzed muscle will be a(n) ____________ squint.

570. yes

571. The amblyoscope will pick up ARC only when it is a well developed constant pattern of seeing. The after-image yields abnormal results for many more types of adaptive seeing.

If you tested 100 cases of esotropia for ARC, would you pick up more cases by using the amblyoscope or the after-image test?

718. central

719. In pleoptics, an ophthalmoscope-like device is always used so that the examiner can see what part of the retina is being used for fixation.

In pleoptic treatment, how does the examiner keep a check on the fixation of the patient?

866. non-

867. A primary concern in orthoptics is thorough evaluation of the binocular status of a patient. Such a work-up would include:

(1) vision testing
(2) squint and phoria analysis
(3) degree of fusion present
(4) type of fixation present
(5) presence of ARC.

In many ways, a preoperative work-up for squint mentioned earlier resembles the above ___________ work-up.

124. *A*

125. A latent strabismus, that is, a deviation of the eyes which is apparent only when both eyes are prevented from looking at the same object, is called a phoria. A latent esotropia is termed an eso ________ .

273. both

274. In the case where an object is presented far to the right, the right eye will be able to get the image on the fovea, but the subject's nose prevents the left eye from seeing the object. Which eye is prevented by the nose from seeing the target *X*?

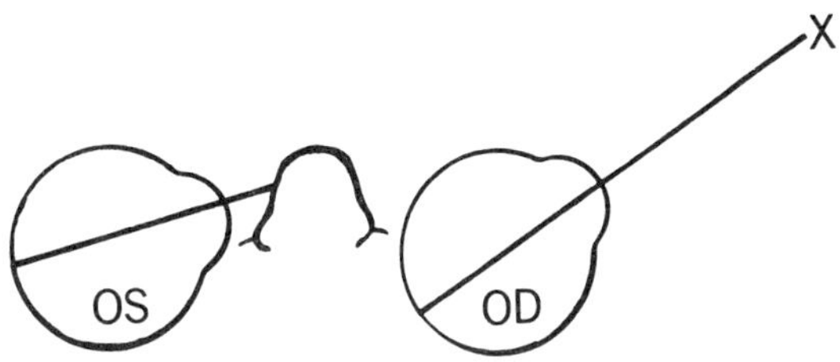

422. incomitant (or noncomitant)

423. The accurate documentation of paralytic squints is helpful in following the improvement which often follows such a paralysis. One measurement is the prism-cover test in the various fields of gaze. Another method is the Lancaster red-green projection test. Two qualitative tests for paralytic squints are the (1) ________ and the (2) ________ .

571. after-image test

572. Because of the fact that the squinting patient may sometimes use both eyes, or may use both eyes in a variety of ways, it is plain that some of our tests will bring out these patterns of seeing and others will not.

Would you expect the after-image test to uncover the same patients with ARC as the amblyoscope?

---

719. by using an ophthalmoscope-like device

720. In pleoptic treatment, the fovea is forced to pick up fixation by one of two methods. In one method, the pseudo fovea is momentarily blinded by a bright light and the real fovea stimulated with different targets.

How is the pseudo fovea prevented from fixating in a pleoptic treatment?

---

867. orthoptic

868. Orthoptics is particularly valuable when fusional reserves, if larger, would afford constantly straight comfortable eyes. Most patients capable of fusion (will/will not) respond to orthoptic exercises with an increase in their fusional reserve.

125. phoria

126. If the patient's dissociated eyes remain on line with the target, he is orthophoric (or said to have orthophoria). The absence of orthophoria is termed heterophoria. Using a Maddox rod to dissociate the eye, the illustrated image would represent ____________.

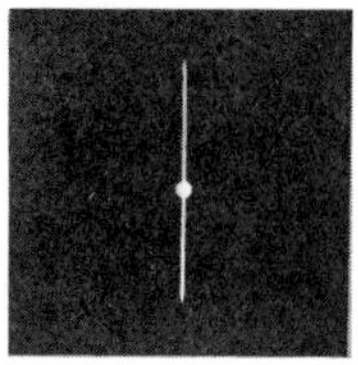

274. OS

275. Although only one eye may be stimulated, both eyes work under the control of the fixation reflex. However, the visual axis of the occluded eye is not always directed at the target if the patient has a phoria or squint.

Under what two conditions does the fixation reflex sometimes fail to bring perfect alignment of the visual axis of the occluded eye?

423. (1) prism-cover test in various fields of gaze
(2) Lancaster red-green projection test
} either order

424. The Lancaster red-green projection test involves the patient wearing red-green glasses. The patient is given a red projector which shines a red light on a screen. If the patient has a red lens over OD and a green lens over OS, he will see the red light with only the ____________.

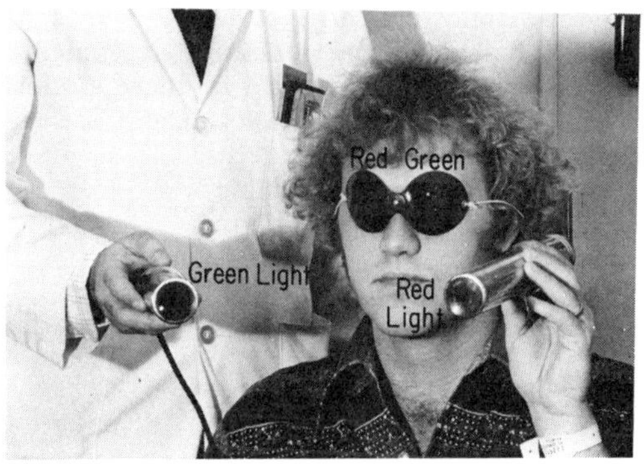

572. no

573. The incidence of constant, well developed ARC in esotropia, using the amblyoscope for testing, is about 50%. However, around 80% of all esotropes may act as if they have ARC in certain test situations.

Before evaluating a study which attempted to get the percentage of ARC in squint cases, what else would you want to know about the study?

720. It is temporarily blinded by a bright light.

721. After many pleoptic sessions, it is hoped that continual blinding of the pseudo fovea and continual use of the real fovea will eventually reestablish foveal fixation.

Does pleoptics reestablish foveal fixation in one session?

868. will

869. The following series of frames shows steps of two basic squint operations, recession and resection. Their techniques are those preferred by one of the authors (RDR). There are many analagous methods which are used to accomplish the same ends, namely weakening or ____________ the muscle a desired amount.

126. orthophoria

127. The absence of orthophoria is termed heterophoria. Thus esophoria, exophoria, and hyperphoria (a latent vertical deviation) are all forms of __________ .

275. (1) phoria } either
(2) squint } order

276. Although only one eye may be stimulated, both eyes usually move. The brain's policy is to coordinate movement of both eyes when any movement is called for.

Is it common for one eye to move while the other remains stationary?

424. OD

425. The examiner performing the Lancaster red-green test shines a projected green light on a screen. If the patient has a red lens over OD and a green lens over OS, he will see the green light with only the __________ .

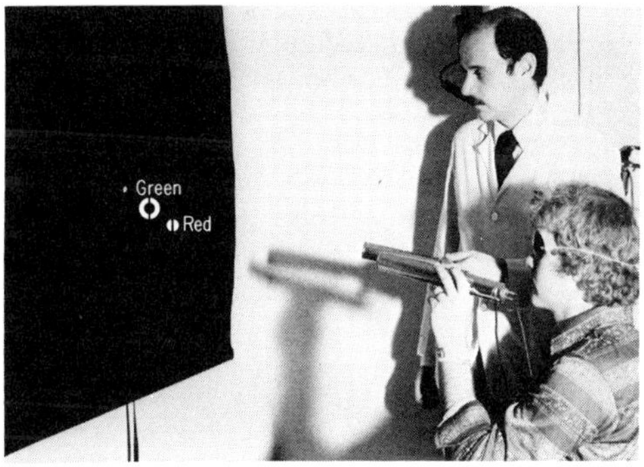

573. the method of testing

574. ARC is much more common in esotropia than in exotropia. This may be related to the fact that the presence of fusion is much more common in exotropia than esotropia. The crude fusion in ARC is not regarded as true fusion.

Is true fusion more common in squints with normal or abnormal retinal correspondence?

---

721. no

722. The other basic pleoptics method momentarily dazzles the area around the real macula. Such a dazzling light induces a ring after-image around the real macula.

What effect does dazzling the area around the real macula have?

---

869. strengthening

870. A recession involves isolating a muscle, severing the muscle's attachment, and ____________ the muscle to the globe at a point posterior to the original insertion.

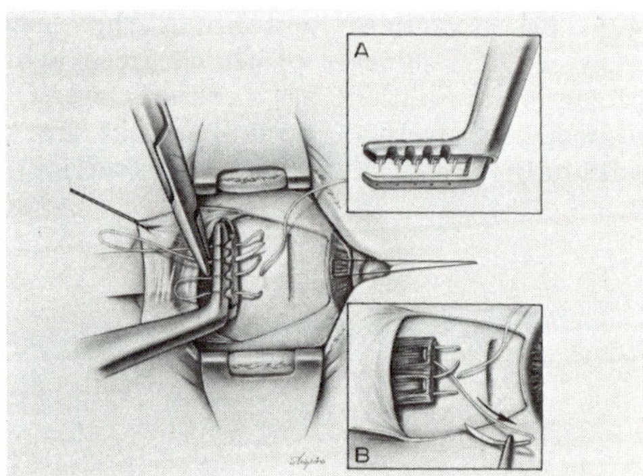

127. heterophoria

128. If one eye deviates nasally, the image will fall on the nasal side of that retina (patient will interpret nasal stimuli as being in the temporal field). The patient will have uncrossed diplopia (right eye sees the right image). The right eye projects its image to which side of the image of the left eye when either eye deviates nasally? (right or left)

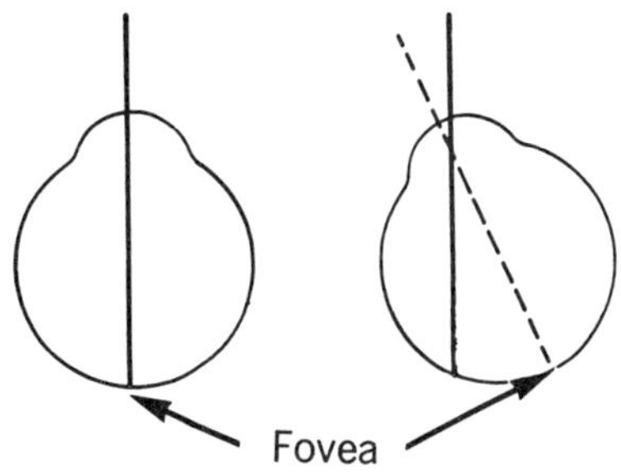

276. no

277. In the diagram, a nonsquinting exophoric subject aligns both visual axes on the target when (both/either/neither) eye(s) is (are) covered.

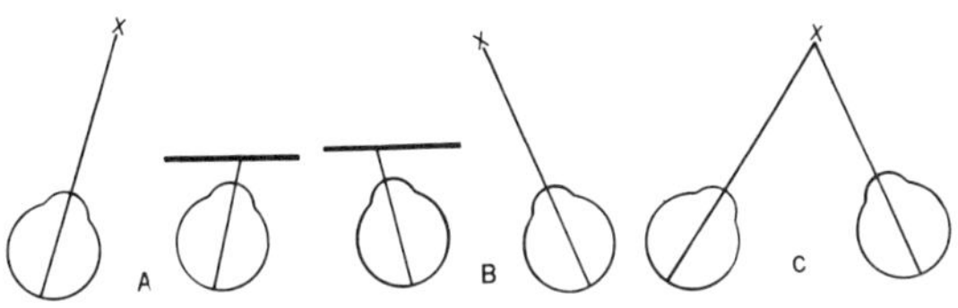

425. OS

426. The examiner using the red-green projection test shines his green light on the screen at any desired point. He asks the patient to superimpose his red light on the green light. The separation of the two lights (as seen by the examiner) on the screen measures the squint. Since each eye of the patient sees its own target, moving the target is like moving a tube of the ________________.
(name of an instrument)

574. normal retinal correspondence

575. The presence of ARC is important in evaluating the prognosis. In a squint case where ARC is present, the chances of achieving fusion after treatment are slight.

How does the presence of abnormal retinal correspondence influence the results of squint treatment?

722. It causes a ring after-image.

723. Once a ring after-image is achieved, the patient is asked to place the ring around smaller and smaller targets.

In pleoptic treatment, what is the patient asked to do with the ring after-image?

870. reattaching (or similar wording)

871. The lateral rectus muscle is to be recessed. The eye is drawn nasally for good exposure. The conjunctiva has been incised and dissected away from the sclera and muscle sheath. Such a conjunctival incision is made initially at the limbus, hence is called a (limbal/fornix) approach.

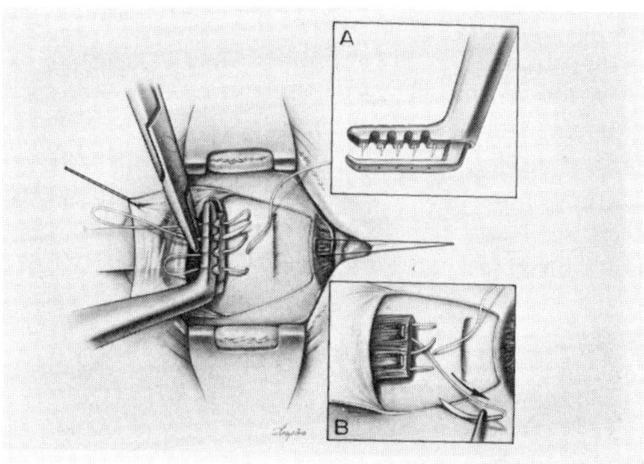

128. right

129. If we have a Maddox rod in front of a right eye which deviates nasally when dissociated, the patient will see <u>(*A*/*B*/*C*)</u>.

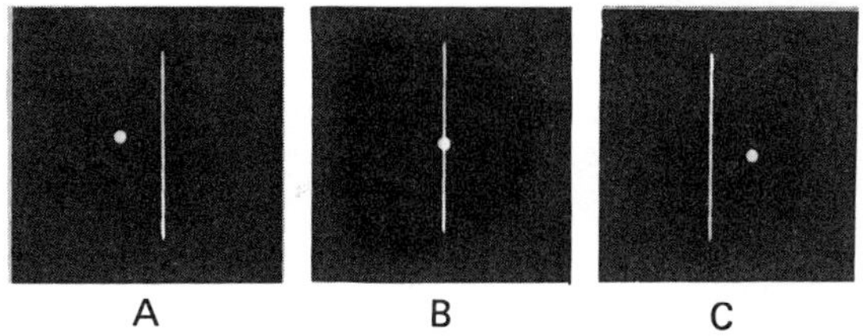

277. neither

278. Although the movements of both eyes are connected, the connection is loose. Perfect alignment of each visual axis is accomplished when both eyes are allowed to receive an image of the target.

Perfect coordination of eye position depends upon visual stimulation of <u>(one/both)</u> eye(s).

426. amblyoscope (or diploscope, haploscope, or synoptophore)

427. Since each eye sees its own target with its fovea, the light of the patient will point in the exact direction the eye is deviating. If the patient has the red lens over OD and is pointing to the left of the green light with his red light, the patient's OD is turned to the <u>(left/right)</u> of his OS. (Remember this is not diplopia, but, like an amblyoscope, the eye is pointing toward the respective light.)

575. The prognosis for fusion development is poor.

576. For a fine grade of fusion, good vision is needed in each eye. Therefore, the prognosis for fusion is poor if the vision in one eye is less than 20/50.

What are the prospects for developing fusion in an esotrope whose vision is: OD 20/20, OS 20/70?

---

723. Place it around smaller and smaller targets.

724. The use of the ring after-image around the real macula forces the patient to learn to fixate with the fovea.

What is the ultimate goal in using the ring after-image?

---

871. limbal

872. The conjunctiva has been incised, dissected away from the muscle, and the intermuscular septum cut permitting a Berens muscle clamp to be applied to the muscle. The muscle has been detached from the globe by severing the muscle at its ____________ .

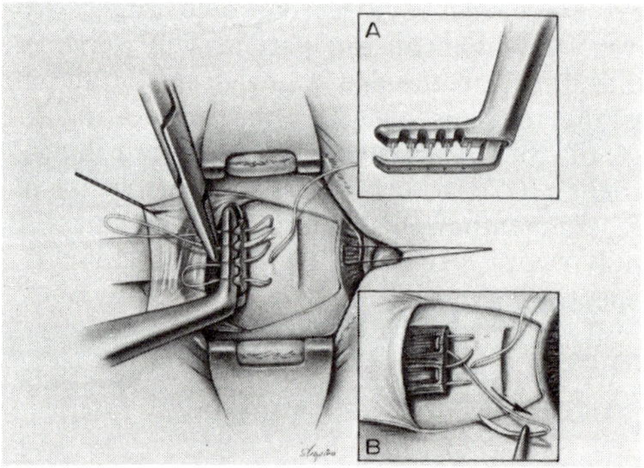

129. *A*

130. If, after dissociation, previously straight eyes now show one eye to be deviated nasally, we call the condition esophoria. If such a patient reports uncrossed diplopia after dissociation, it is confirmation of his ____________.

---

278. both

279. The eye behind the cover (in a nonsquinter) may remain directed toward the target, it might turn out, or it might turn in. Once the cover is removed, and the eye receives visual stimulation, it aligns properly.

If an eye of a nonsquinting subject turns out behind a cover, will it turn in to the target when the cover is removed?

---

427. left

428. The screen for the Lancaster red-green projection test is calibrated in 2° squares. If the patient has a red lens over OD and points 6 squares to the left of zero while the examiner points to zero with the green light, the patient has (1) ____________$^{\circ}$ (2) ____________.

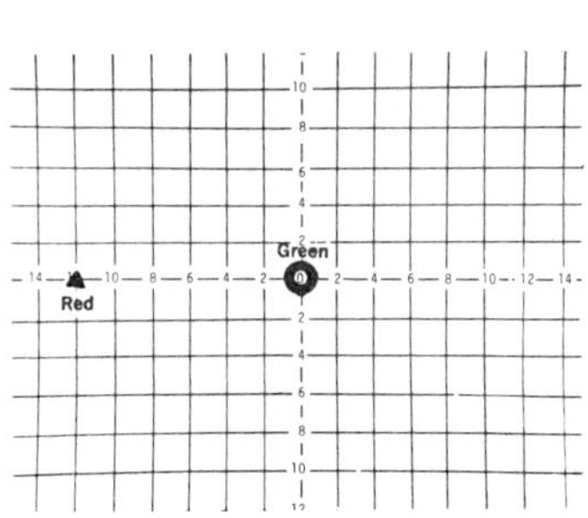

576. poor

577. When an eye not only turns in (esotropia) or out (exotropia) but also deviates vertically (turns up or down), the prognosis for fusion is worse than if no vertical deviation was present.

How does the addition of a vertical turn to a horizontal deviation affect prognosis for fusion?

724. foveal fixation

725. It is generally felt that if the amblyope shows no improvement after about ten pleoptic sessions, then the prognosis is very poor.

How many sessions of pleoptics should be given before one gets an idea of whether the treatment will be beneficial?

872. insertion

873. The Berens clamp is designed to permit a firm grasp of the tissue, while holes in the clamp allow the needle to be ___________.

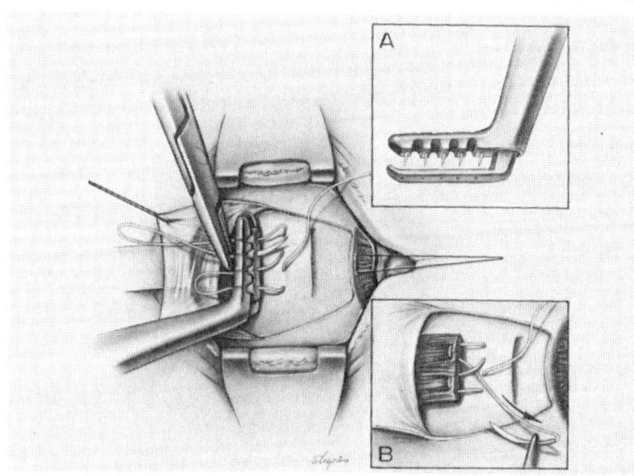

130. esophoria

131. If the dissociated eye deviates temporally, the image will fall on the temporal side of the retina (which will be interpreted as being nasal), and crossed diplopia will be reported. If the right eye deviates temporally, it projects its image to which side of the image of the left eye?

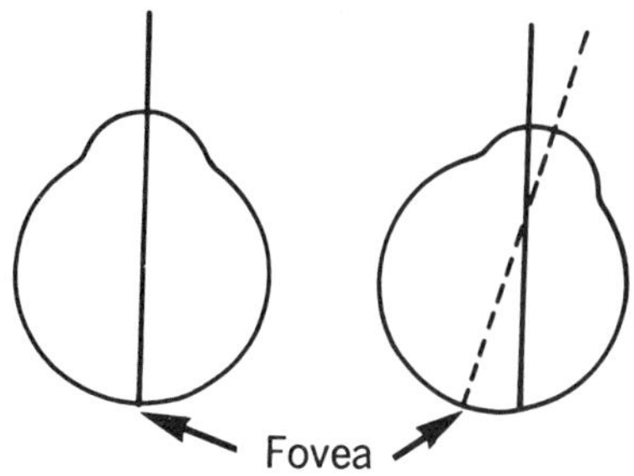

279. yes

280. We consider an eye which deviates behind a cover as having a tendency to squint. If the eye turns out, it is called an exo tendency; if the eye turns in, it is called an eso tendency.

How is the tendency to squint in a nonsquinting patient determined?

428. (1) 12
(2) esotropia (or esophoria)

429. The squares on the Lancaster screen are faintly marked so the patient sees only the red light with one eye and the green light with the other. The patient superimposes the green light on the red light. The patient sees (1) <u>(*A*/*B*)</u>, and the examiner sees (2) <u>(*A*/*B*)</u>.

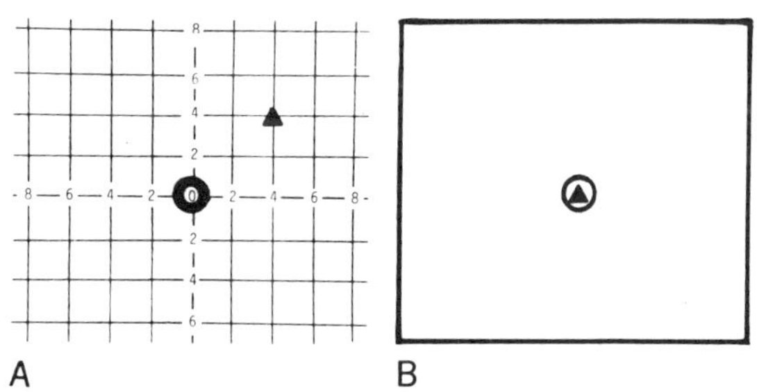

577. makes it worse

578. It is obvious that many factors influence the prognosis for fusion after treatment in a case of squint.

List five of the seven factors in cases of esotropia which tend to improve the prognosis for fusion.

725. ten

726. Once pleoptic treatment is started in earnest, maximum benefit should come in four to five months.

How long is pleoptic treatment usually continued?

873. imbricated in the muscle (or similar wording)

874. By tracing the path of the applied suture, you can identify a "figure of eight" design. The scleral bites are made (perpendicular/parallel) to the limbus.

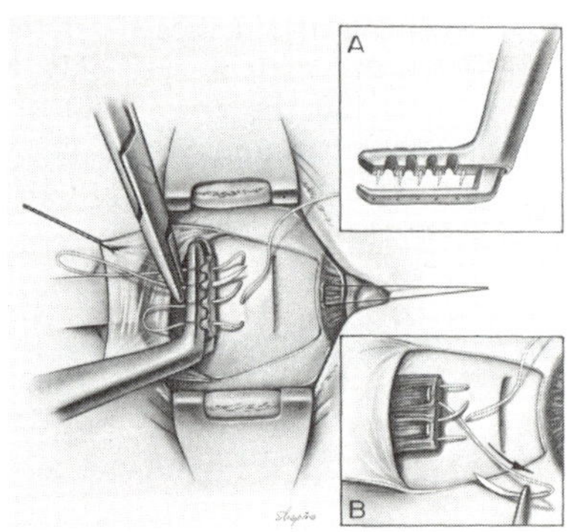

131. left

132. The turning temporally of a dissociated eye is termed exophoria. Crossed diplopia, as reported by a patient after dissociation, implies he has ______________.

280. During fixation, cover one eye and note whether it deviates and the direction of deviation.

281. This tendency for the visual axis of the covered eye to bear to one side or the other is called a **phoria**, derived from the Greek word meaning "to bear."

An exophoria describes the tendency of the covered eye to (1) ______________.

An esophoria describes the tendency of the covered eye to (2) ______________.

Orthophoria describes the condition in which the covered eye (3) ______________.

429. (1) *B*
(2) *A*

430. To quantitate a paralytic squint, the examiner shines his light in the various fields of gaze. If the patient has an incomitant squint, the separation of the lights (to the examiner) will ______________ in the different fields of gaze.

578. (1) fully accommodative esotropia
(2) no ARC
(3) good vision OU
(4) no vertical component
(5) presence of pretreatment fusion
(6) late onset
(7) intermittency
(any five)

579. A number of factors are also involved in the prognosis for fusion in exotropia.

List four factors which may favorably influence the prognosis for fusion in exotropia.

726. four to five months

727. About 40% of the cases of eccentric fixation respond successfully to pleoptic treatment.

In a group of 100 eccentric fixators, how many will respond to pleoptic treatment?

874. parallel

875. The amount of recession is determined by the scleral bites. A caliper setting of 8 mm would measure 8 mm from the original insertion to the __________.

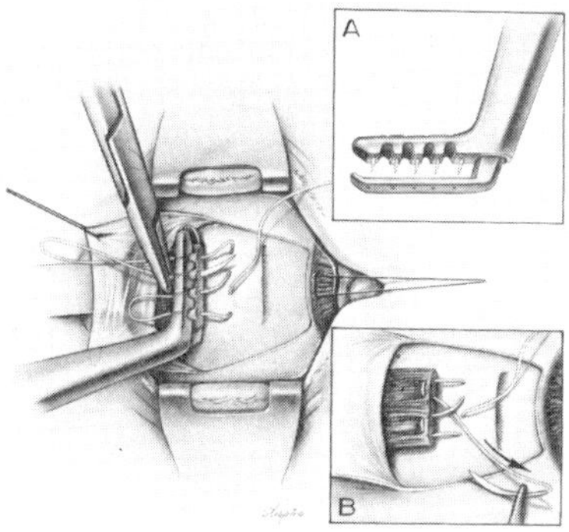

132. exophoria

133. After dissociation with a Maddox rod OD, the patient with exophoria reports (*A/B/C*).

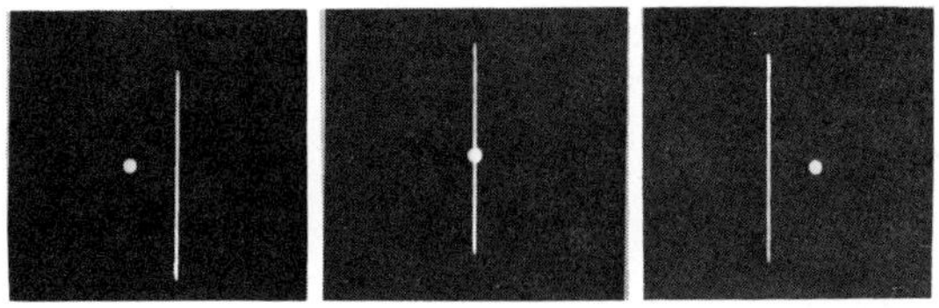

A B C

281. (1) turn out
(2) turn in
(3) does not deviate

282. To determine the type of phoria, you may either see which way the eye deviates behind the cover or wait until the cover is removed and see which way the eye turns to pick up fixation.

If an eye turns in behind a cover, which way will it turn when the cover is removed?

430. vary

431. Each eye has a medial and lateral rectus muscle which is responsible for moving the eye from side to side. To look to the right, as in the photo, the patient uses the right (1) ____________ muscle and the left (2) ____________ muscle.

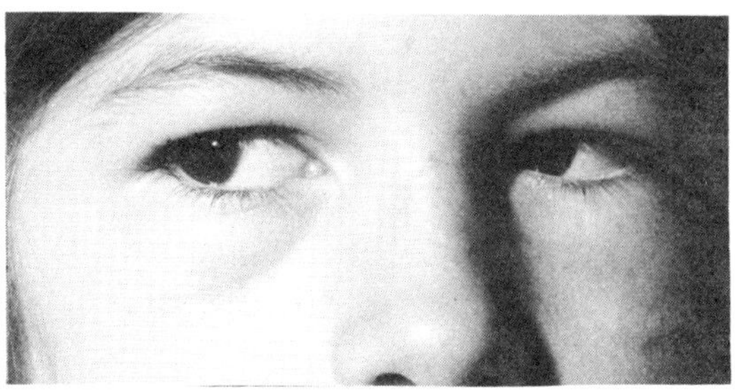

579. (1) good vision OU (2) squint under 20 prism diopters (3) presence of pretreatment fusion (4) no ARC (5) no vertical component (6) intermittency (any four)

580. While 85% of exotropes have intermittent fusion, the overall prognosis for constant fusion and straight eyes of exotropes after treatment is about 60%.

In a group of 100 cases of exotropia, how many would have constant fusion and be straight after treatment?

---

727. about 40

728. Pleoptics is also used in cases of central fixation amblyopia which do not respond to patching.

Aside from eccentric fixation, when else is pleoptic treatment used?

---

875. scleral bites

876. The "figure of eight" technique depends upon ____________ knot(s), hence the suture used should be strong and the knot should not slip.

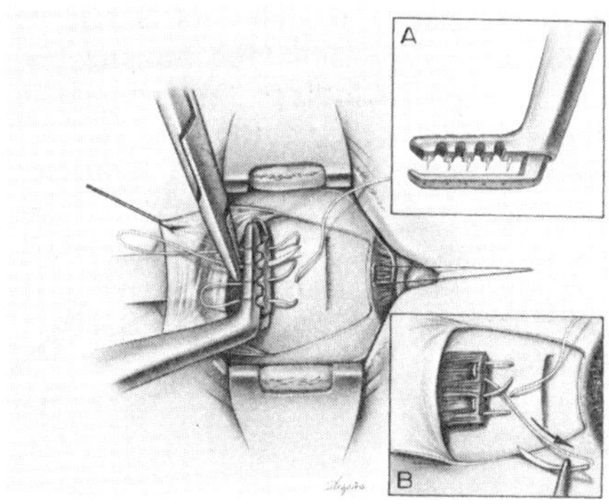

133. *C*

134. The deviations of the dissociated eye nasally or temporally are termed **horizontal phorias.** Vertical phorias do exist and should be checked. Rotation of the dissociating Maddox rod to the vertical position permits this measurement and causes the patient to see a horizontal line. In the absence of vertical phoria (vertical orthophoria), the patient sees (*A*/*B*/*C*).

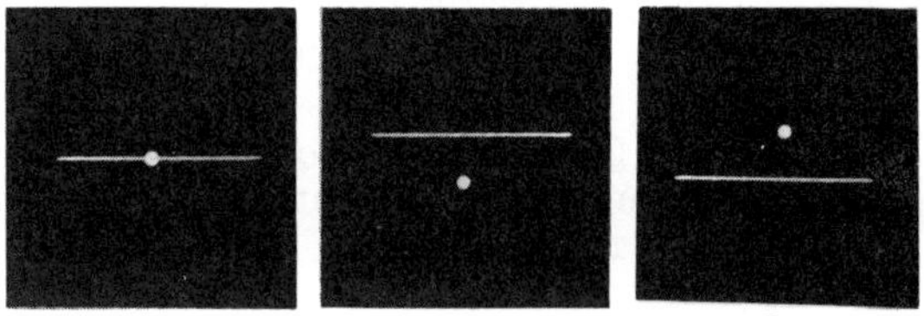

A B C

282. out

283. The normal range for phorias in distance viewing is from orthophoria to 4 prism diopters of exophoria.

If an eye turns back in 4 prism diopters upon removal of the cover:

(1) What type of phoria is it?
(2) How much is the phoria?
(3) Is it in the normal range?

431. (1) lateral rectus
(2) medial rectus

432. Eye muscles that move the eyes in the same direction are called **yoke muscles.** The right medial rectus muscle is a yoke muscle of the left ______________ muscle since each muscle moves its eye to the left.

580. 60

581. The overall prognosis for constant fusion in esotropia is poorer than for exotropia. Of a large group of esotropes which included all the variations, about one-third have constant fusion after treatment.

In a group of 100 cases of esotropia of all types, how many would have constant fusion and be straight after treatment?

---

728. in cases of amblyopia unresponsive to patching

729. Pleoptics helps restore vision in about ____________% of centrally fixating amblyopes who do not respond to patching.

(*See Table 1 preceding the index.*)

---

876. one

877. A nonabsorbable suture is often used with this technique, thus the knot should be hidden under the muscle end to prevent its being seen under the conjunctiva. Insert B shows the final path of the needle (under/over) the earlier path to allow the knot to be tucked under the muscle end.

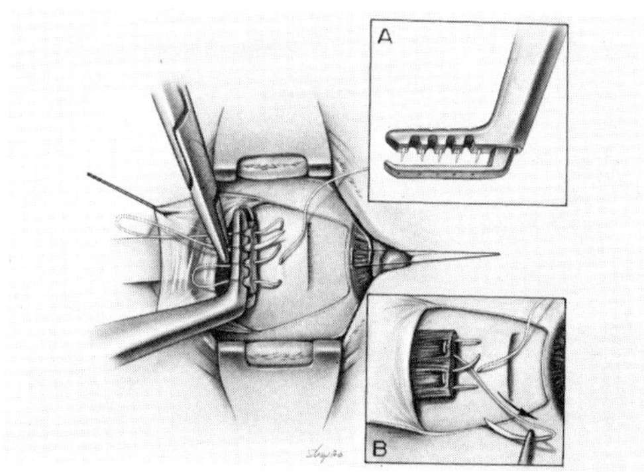

134. *A*

135. Phorias may be measured by dissociating the eyes by a Maddox rod and adding prisms to align the images. A patient fixates on a light while having a Maddox rod in front of OD and sees the images as depicted in diagram *A*. A prism base (nasal/temporal) will be necessary to align the images as depicted by diagram *B*. (Remember a prism displaces an image toward its apex.)

A B

283. (1) exophoria
(2) 4 prism diopters
(3) yes

284. A detailed target is used for near phoria testing to encourage accommodation for sharp focusing. Accommodation brings in convergence, and so the test approximates the condition of the eyes during reading or sewing.

Would you expect the eye behind the cover during a near phoria test to turn in more or less if a watch, as opposed to a light, were used as the target?

432. lateral rectus

433. The right lateral rectus muscle moves the right eye to the right. The left medial rectus moves the left eye to the right. This means that the right lateral rectus muscle is a ______________ muscle of the left medial rectus muscle.

581. 33

582. The prognosis for good cosmetic results varies directly with the number of operations performed—the more operations the better the chances of a good result.

If an esotrope is not cosmetically straight after one operation, would you advise a second operation? (1)__________ Why? (2)__________ .

729. 50

730. The equipment used for pleoptic training is expensive, and the sessions are daily or thrice weekly. Comparative studies have cast doubt on whether pleoptic training really cures patients who will not respond to other treatment. Is the worth of pleoptics proven?

877. under

878. Excessive scarring results from poor attention to hemostasis, sloppy dissection, and suture reactions. A benefit of nonabsorbable sutures is the lack of __________ .

135. temporal

136. If a prism base is temporal before an eye, we call the prism direction base-out. If the prism base is nasal, we call the prism direction base-__________.

284. more

285. In testing the phoria for near, ask the patient to view a detailed target (a watch or a card with symbols) and alternately cover one eye, then the other.

Is a flashlight a good target for near phoria testing?

433. yoke

434. The yoke muscle of the left medial rectus muscle is the (1)__________ muscle, since each muscle moves its eye to the (2)__________.

582. (1) yes
(2) The prognosis for cosmetic cure gets better with each operation.

583. About 60% of all esotropes will appear straight after one operation. After two operations, about 80% of the remaining esotropes will be cosmetically straight. After one unsuccessful operation an esotrope stands a (4:1/3:1) chance of being straight after the next operation.

730. no

731. Comparative studies of pleoptics vs. patching and use of red filter have indicated that pleoptics may not have any advantages over the latter. The disadvantages of pleoptics are: (1) ____________ and (2) ____________ .

878. suture reaction

879. In general, the smaller the suture used, the less the reaction. In the selection of the suture, you would select the smallest diameter consistent with the strength needed with your ____________ .

136. in

137. Esophoria (uncrossed diplopia) is measured with prism base-__________.

285. no

286. The normal range of phorias during near viewing is orthophoria to 6 prism diopters of exophoria.

If a near phoria is 5 prism diopters of exophoria when looking at a flashlight target, it would probably be (1) __________ than 5 prism diopters of exophoria when looking at some small print. If the near phoria, while using fine print as a target, is 8 prism diopters exophoria, is it in the normal range? (2) __________.

434. (1) right lateral rectus
(2) right

435. The photo demonstrates the patient using the yoke muscles consisting of the (1)__________ and (2)__________.

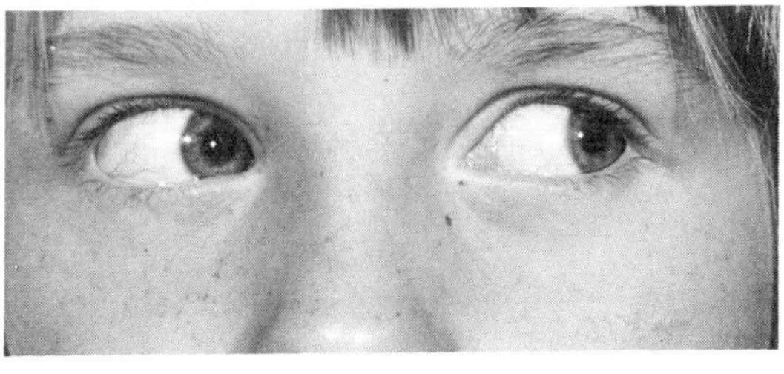

583. 4:1

584.

PART VIII
ETIOLOGY

(Advance to next frame.)

731. (1) cost and time
(2) questionable advantage over simpler methods

732. It must be appreciated that once vision is restored in the amblyopic eye, conditions which caused the original suppression must be corrected.

If amblyopia is corrected in a deviated eye, and nothing is done to correct the squint, will the amblyopia return?

879. technique

880. After tightening and tying the suture, subsequent to the step shown in B, the knot is tucked under the muscle end, the conjunctival incision is closed and the operation known as ____________ is complete.

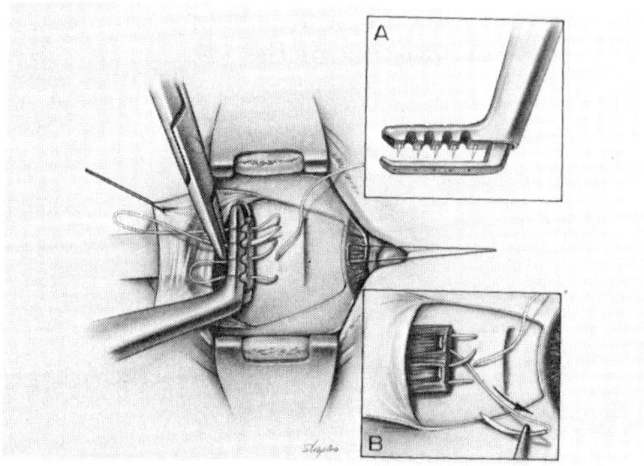

137. out

138. Exophoria (crossed diplopia) is measured with prism base-__________ .

286. (1) less
(2) no

287. When the fixating eye is covered in a patient with exotropia, it will turn out. However, what is more important is that the deviating eye will turn in to pick up fixation.

If the fixating eye is covered in a patient with an exotropia, which way will each eye shift?

435. (1) left lateral rectus } either
(2) right medial rectus } order

436. Four muscles are responsible for elevation and depression of each eye. When the eye is directed temporally 25°, the superior rectus elevates, and the inferior rectus __________ the eye.

584. *(Advance to next frame.)*

585. Before reviewing the various theories concerned with the cause of squint, let us review the chain of events preceding an eye movement. At first, the eyes become aware of something in space that should be investigated.

Before most eye movements start, a(n) ____________ on the retina is noted.

732. yes

733. Improvement from pleoptic training may not be lasting even in patients who have good fusion.

Is the presence of good fusion a guarantee that visual improvement after pleoptic training will be permanent?

880. recession

881. Resection of an extraocular muscle involves (1) ____________ a distal portion of the muscle and suturing the muscle back to the original insertion site, thus (2) ____________ the muscle.

The following frames show the resection operation.

138. in

139. An easy way to remember that exophoria produces crossed diplopia when the images are dissociated is to remember that there is an *X* (or cross) in exophoria. A result of exophoria is ______________ diplopia after dissociation.

287. The covered eye will deviate out; the other eye will turn in to fixate on the target.

288. In patients with phorias, only the eye behind the cover shifts. The exception is in orthophoria, when neither eye shifts.

In a case of esophoria, what happens to each eye when the left eye is covered (just prior to the covering of the left eye, both eyes were uncovered)?

436. depresses

437. When the eye is turned in about 50°, the obliques elevate and depress. The obliques insert on the back of the eye and pull forward, so the superior oblique pulls the eye down and the inferior oblique pulls the eye ______________.

585. image (or stimulus)

586. The retinal image is then encoded and, in the form of a nerve message, is sent to the visual cortex for interpretation.

The retina takes the information from the image and ____________ it before sending the report to the brain.

733. no

734. A child occasionally will successfully resist all attempts to patch his good eye. Penalization is a technique which may be useful in such a patient. The technique has variations, but is based upon the monocular use of atropine in the good eye. If the good eye is hyperopic, the atropine will blur that eye at distance and the blur from the atropine at near in such an eye will be (slight/severe).

881. (1) excising (or removing) } or similar wording
(2) shortening (or strengthening)

882. The OD is pulled ____________ to approach and resect the medial rectus.

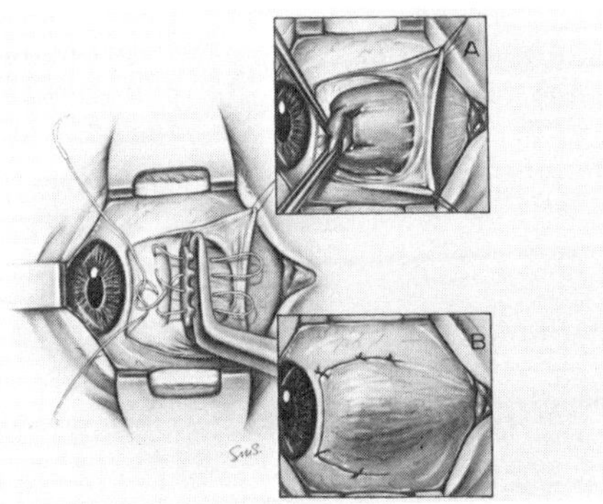

139. crossed

140. Revolving prisms provide an easy method of increasing or decreasing the prisms used to measure phorias. Prisms placed apex to base, if of equal power, provide no prismatic power. If prism *A* is rotated in relation to prism *B*, the neutralizing value of *A* is reduced, and a measurable prismatic effect is gained. If prism *A* is changed from the diagram and placed apex to apex with prism *B*, then the total prismatic power is _____________.

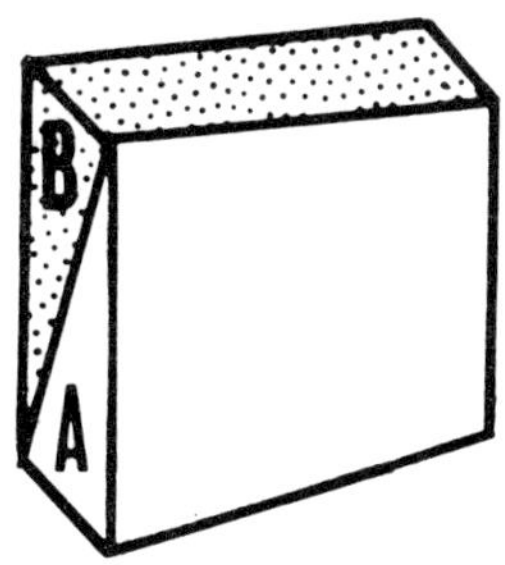

288. left eye turns in
right eye stays fixed to target

289. In patients with squints, either both eyes shift if the fixating eye is covered, or both remain stationary if the deviating eye is covered.

Describe the movement of both eyes if the fixating eye is covered in a case of exotropia.

437. up

438. The yoke muscle of the right superior oblique is the _____________ muscle which moves the left eye down when the eyes are looking to the left.

586. encodes (or processes)

587. Once the message is interpreted, a plan is brought forth which will best move both eyes into a position where the most sensitive parts of both retinas can analyze the target.

What is the advantage of directing the foveas at a new object?

734. severe

735. The atropine should be applied to the good eye two times per week. After several weeks of the penalization therapy a child may tolerate patching. Failure of parents to patch a child usually indicates a trial of ____________ .

882. temporally (or to the right, or laterally)

883. The conjunctival incision shown is called the ____________ approach.

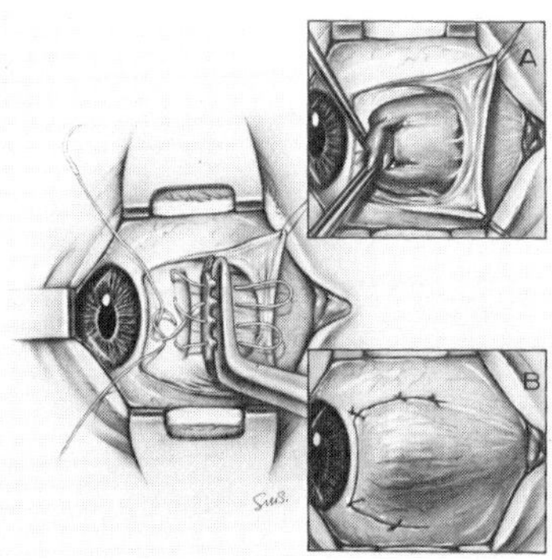

140. power of prism *A* plus power of prism *B*

. . . .

141. Measurement of heterophoria is necessary. The phoria may be conveniently measured with prisms. With the Maddox rod in front of OD, the patient sees *A*. A prism displaces an image toward its apex. A suitable amount of prism base- (in/out) OS will change the picture to *B*.

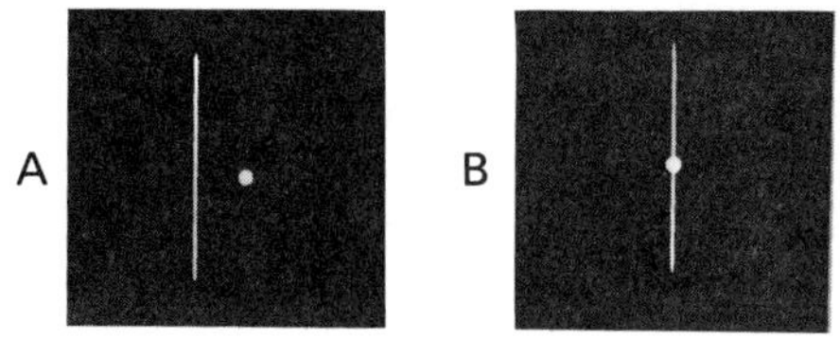

---

289. The deviating eye turns in to pick up fixation and the fixating eye turns out behind the cover.

. . . .

290. The type of refractive error in a group of exotropes does not vary from the pattern of refractive errors seen in a group of nonsquinting subjects.

If the average refractive error is a moderate amount of farsightedness in a group of nonsquinting children, what is the average refractive error in a similar age group of exotropic children?

---

438. left inferior rectus

. . . .

439. The yoke muscle of the right inferior oblique is the ____________ muscle which moves the left eye up when the eyes are looking to the left.

587. They are able to record more information about the target (or similar wording).

588. Since the plan for eye movements involves coordinated, well timed contractions of all the eye muscles, messages are now sent along nerves to the eye muscles.

In order to accomplish a smooth eye movement, some muscles ____________ , while others contract, and some help steady the eye during movement.

735. penalization (or atropine)

736.

PART X
TREATMENT OF SQUINTS

(Advance to next frame.)

883. limbal

884. The suturing technique shown is basically the same as that shown in the recession procedure and is called the ____________ technique.

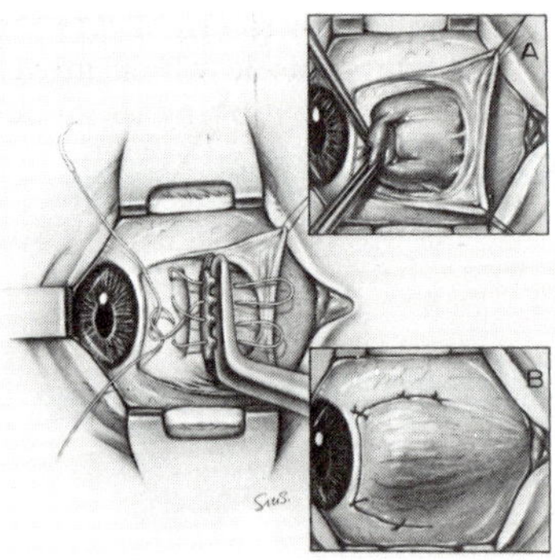

141. in

142. You will remember that if a prism is placed so that its base is temporal, we refer to this as prism base-out; if nasal, prism base- (1) ____________ .

Prism base-out measures esophoria. Prism base- (2) ____________ measures exophoria.

290. a moderate amount of farsightedness

291. Although both eyes do not work together in exotropia, the vision in each eye, tested separately, is usually good.

Is it common to find a vision of 20/20 in each eye in an exotrope?

439. left superior rectus

440. The patient in the photo is using the right superior rectus muscle and its yoke muscle, the left ____________ muscle.

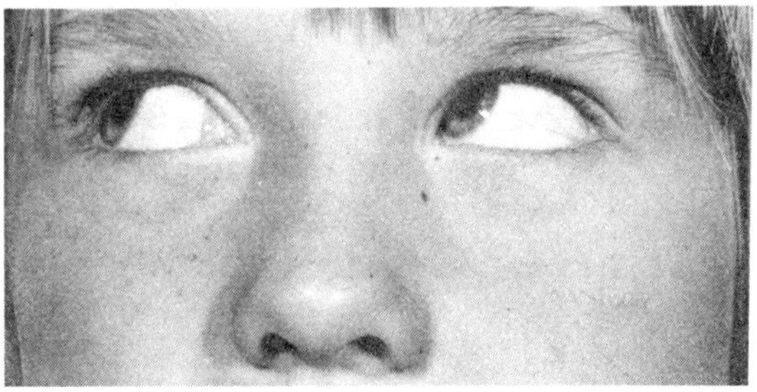

588. relax

589. A fusion control in the brain supervises the movement of both eyes so that the eventual retinal image will fall on corresponding retinal areas, providing a reflex fusional movement.

Since the eyes move in a reflex manner to receive a retinal image on corresponding areas without the conscious effort of the subject, the ________ movement might be considered reflex in nature.

736. (*Advance to next frame.*)

737. About 10% of all esotropes are cured without surgery. These represent the fully accommodative type. Of exotropes, only a small percentage respond to other than surgical treatment.

What is the most common means of successfully treating squint?

884. figure of eight

885. The amount of muscle to be resected is measured from the (1) ________ to the applied (2) ________.

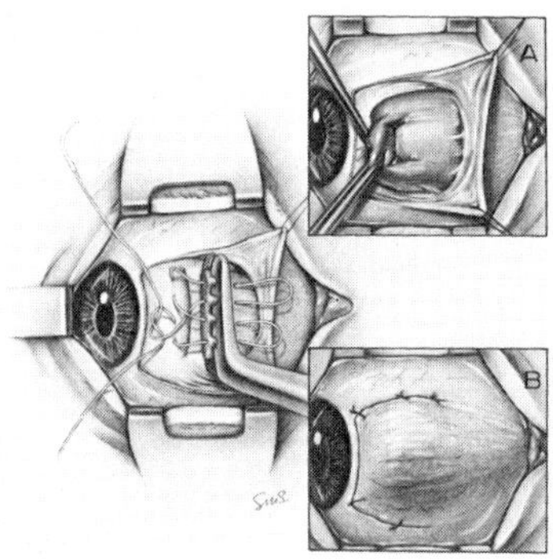

142. (1) in
(2) in

143. Revolving prisms are commercially available and appear as indicated. The figures and line indicate the prism diopters and base of the prism. In the photo, the patient reports the targets aligned and thus has (1) ____________ △ (2) ____________ phoria.

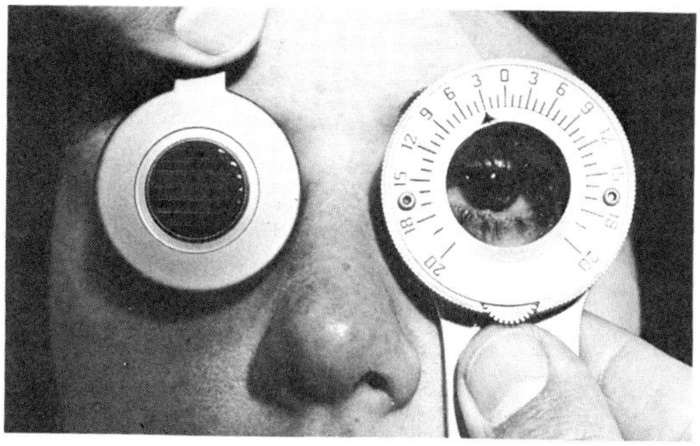

291. yes

292. Often, the exotrope complains of increased sensitivity to bright lights (photophobia). This may be based on a difficulty in suppressing one image in bright light.

The symptom of photophobia in an exotrope may be due to ____________.

440. inferior oblique

441. The right medial rectus and the left lateral rectus muscles are examples of (1) ____________, which cause the eyes to look to the (2) ____________ when innervated.

589. fusional

590. It is generally felt that in squint the trouble lies either: (a) in the coordinating system of the brain; (b) in the nerve going to the muscles; or (c) in the muscle or its ligaments and tendons. The nerve can be incriminated in muscle paralysis.

If the medial rectus was paralyzed, causing an exotropia, where would the lesion probably be?

737. surgery

738. Accommodative esotropes may be corrected with plus lenses, since by definition their esotropia is due to too much convergence for a fixed amount of ____________ .

885. (1) insertion
(2) Berens (muscle) clamp

886. Careful attention in the application of the muscle clamp is important in any muscle operation to avoid the muscle's slipping from the clamp and retracting to ____________ .

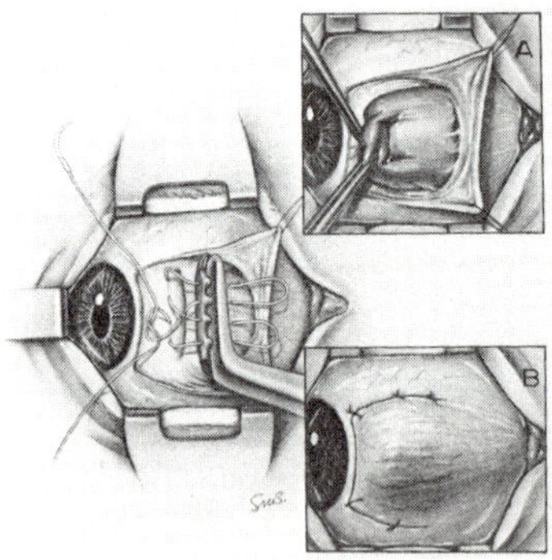

143. (1) 3
(2) exo

144. The zero on the revolving prism is placed at 90° to measure horizontal deviations. As the line is moved in, base-in is indicated, and as the indicator line is moved out, base- (1) ____________ is indicated.

The photo indicates an exophoria of (2) ____________ △.

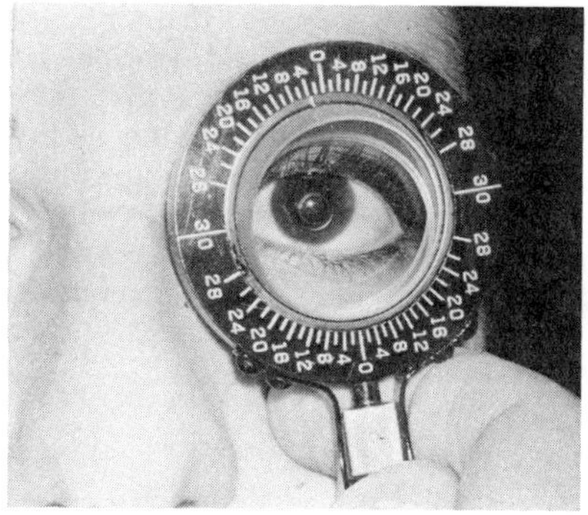

292. the difficulty in suppressing one image in bright light (or diplopia in bright light)

293.

PART IV
ESOTROPIA

(Advance to next frame.)

441. (1) yoke muscles
(2) left

442. The yoke muscle of the right inferior rectus is the (1) ____________ . The yoke muscle of the left superior rectus is the (2) ____________ .

590. the nerve

591. Impairment of any one of a number of brain functions has been suggested as the cause of squint. For example, many feel that the ability of the brain to direct corresponding retinal areas to a target and then unify the impressions from each retina (fusion) is at fault in squint. Fusion impairment is more common in esotropia than in exotropia. Esotropes would be considered to have a dysfunction of the ____________, causing inability to fuse.

738. accommodation (or hyperopia)

739. A cycloplegic refraction with atropine or a combination of proparacaine, cyclopentolate, and tropicamide is necessary to determine all the hyperopia in esotropia. If plus lenses straighten the eyes, the esotropia is entirely ____________ .

886. the back of the orbit (or similar wording)

887. The suture is placed at the ____________ in the resection operation.

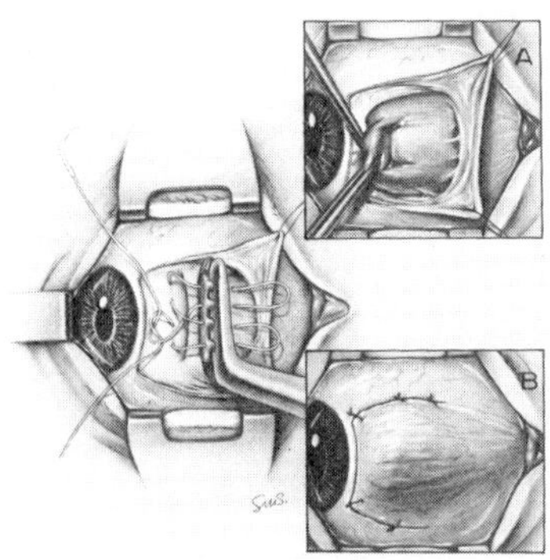

144. (1) out
(2) 4

145. With the Maddox rod over one eye, and the revolving prism in front of the other, prismatic power is increased in the proper direction until the patient reports the light to be on the line. If the patient sees *A* (with Maddox rod OD), the patient has (1) ____________ phoria, and prism base- (2) ____________ must be used for measurement.

A

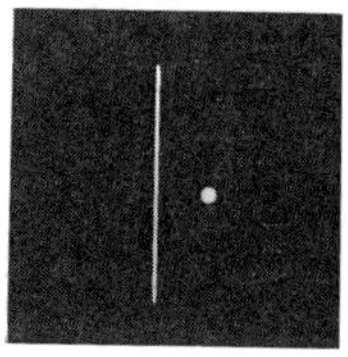

293. (*Advance to next frame.*)

294. Approximately 80% of all squint cases have esotropia.

(1) Given 100 cases of strabismus, how many would you expect to have crossed eyes?

(2) How many would you expect to have exotropia?

442. (1) left superior oblique
(2) right inferior oblique

443. The diagram summarizes the yoke muscles. Each pair of arrows which are parallel and in the same direction represents yoke muscles. The right inferior oblique (IO) is the yoke muscle of the left ____________ .

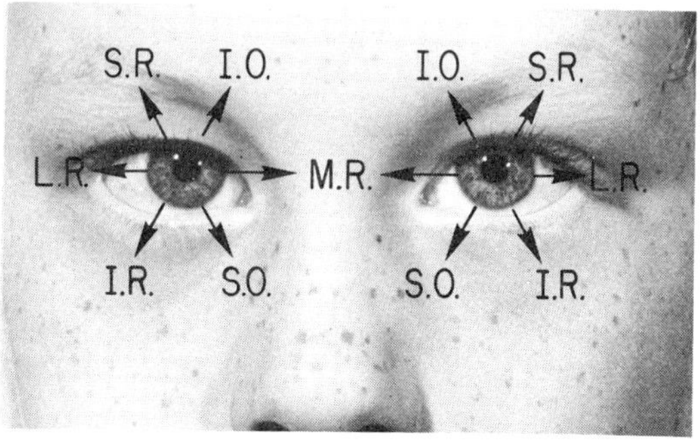

591. brain (fusion center)

592. Studies have shown that although squints may run in families, defects in fusion do not run in families. (An exception to this rule may be the stereoblind.)

Is poor fusion generally thought to be inherited in the squinting patient?

739. accommodative

740. If any portion of an esotropia is accommodative, that part should not be corrected with surgery. Nonaccommodative esotropia is usually a (1) ____________ problem, and accommodative esotropia is usually a (2) ____________ problem.

887. original insertion

888. The insert A shows the suture knot and ends being tucked ____________ to prevent its later visibility.

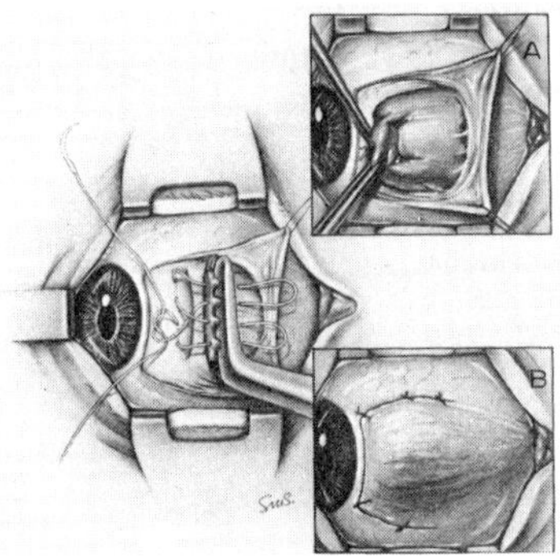

145. (1) exo
(2) in

146. If the patient sees *A* (with Maddox rod OD), he has (1) ____________ phoria which can be measured by adding prism base- (2) ____________ .

A

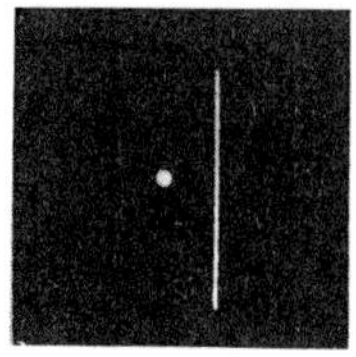

294. (1) 80
(2) 20

295. Accommodation is linked to convergence of the eyes.

(1) If a subject changes fixation from a distant object to the print on a page, does he accommodate?

(2) Does he converge?

443. superior rectus (SR)

444. The photo demonstrates the patient using the (1) ____________ muscle and its yoke muscle, the (2) ____________ .

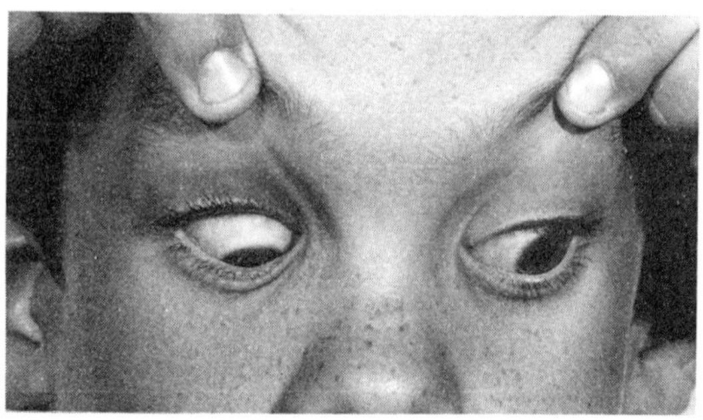

592. no

593. Fusion is not an inherited faculty, but one develops it at an early age. Some squinters are blocked from properly learning fusion. Fusion is considered not to be (1) ____________ , but the patient may not (2) ____________ the fusion properly at an early age.

740. (1) surgical
(2) nonsurgical (or refraction)

741. Any hyperopia +.75 or over detected in a cycloplegic refraction should be given for the esotrope to wear so that the ____________ portion of the esotropia can be determined.

888. under the muscle end

889. The insert B shows closure of the conjunctiva with Black 0000000 silk ____________ sutures. These interrupted sutures fall out by themselves in seven to ten days.

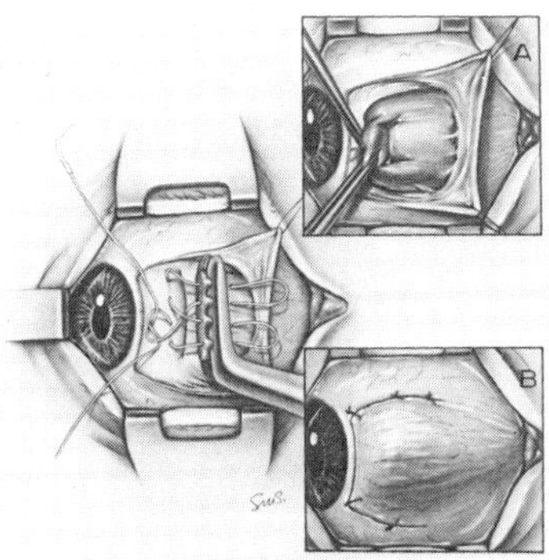

146. (1) eso
(2) out

147. Vertical phorias are denoted by the eye which is higher in the dissociated state. The eye which is higher is termed hyperphoric. If the right eye is higher, the patient has a right hyperphoria. If the right eye is lower, the patient has a ____________ .

295. (1) yes
(2) yes

296. The accommodative convergence/accommodation ratio (ACA ratio) for a specific individual means that when he accommodates a certain amount, he automatically converges a set amount. One diopter of accommodation for a specific individual will always elicit (the same/variable) amount of convergence.

444. (1) left inferior rectus } either
(2) right superior oblique } order

445. The patient in the photo is using the (1) ____________ muscle and its yoke muscle, the (2) ____________ .

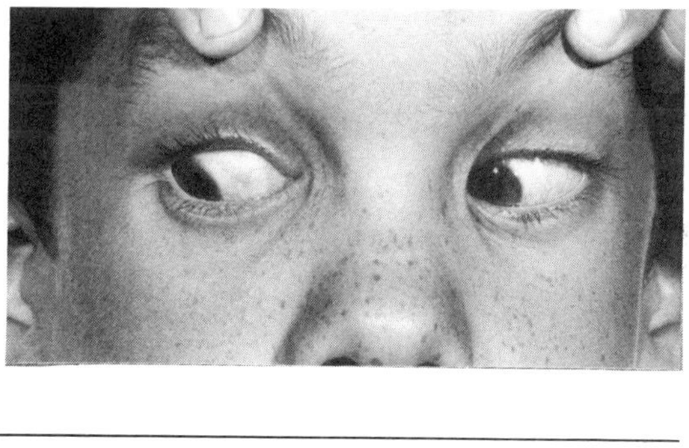

593. (1) inherited
(2) develop

594. Although poor fusion is not inherited, obstacles in the development of the fusional process could exist. For example, if one eye of a child becomes blind, the child will often develop a squint.

Unilateral blindness interferes with the development of fusion since the brain receives only ____________ image.

741. accommodative (or nonaccommodative)

742. If the plus lenses correct an esotropia at distance, but the patient is still esotropic at near, you would suspect him to have a (high/low) ACA.

889. interrupted

890. Closure of the conjunctiva completes the medial rectus strengthening procedure known as ____________ .

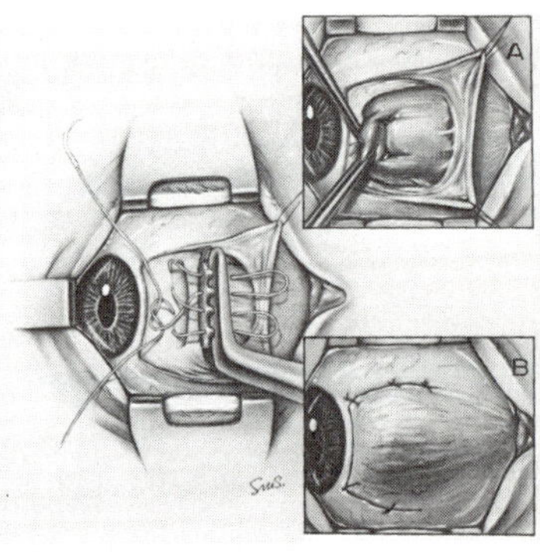

147. left hyperphoria

148. When one eye deviates upward, while the other eye remains aligned on a target, the image of the target will fall on the upper portion of the retina of the deviating eye and remain on the fovea of the fixating eye. What portion of the retina of the downward deviating eye will be stimulated while the other eye fixates a target? (upper/lower)

---

296. the same

297. An individual's ACA ratio is inherited and is constant for that individual.

Would identical twins have the same ACA ratio?

---

445. (1) left superior oblique } either
(2) right inferior rectus } order

446. The patient in the photo is using the (1) ____________ muscle and its yoke muscle, the (2) ____________ .

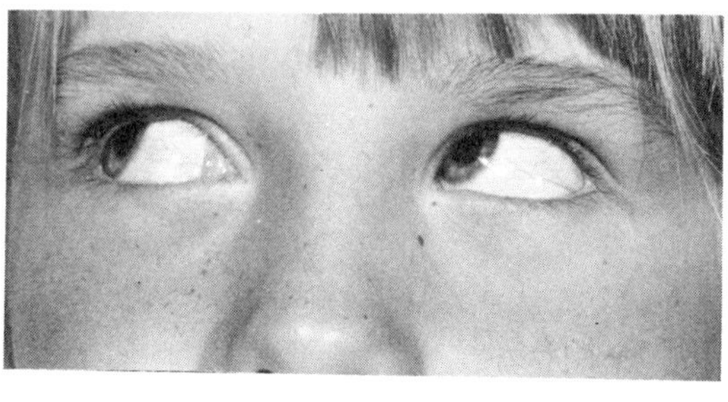

594. one

595. A useful relationship between the age of onset of unilateral blindness to the presence or absence of an XT or ET is the following:

1) Unilateral congenitally blind eye typically gives straight eyes.

2) A child age one to six years developing a unilateral blind eye commonly develops an esotropia.

3) Onset of unilateral blindness from age 7 to 11 often permits straight eyes.

4) Unilateral blindness after age twelve typically gives an exotropia.

From the above you could generalize that the older the child at the onset of unilateral blindness the better the chance for __________ .

(RETURN TO PAGE 2 FOR ANSWER 595.)

742. high

743. Since the esotrope who is straight for distance but esotropic for near has a high ACA ratio, additional plus for near may make his esotropia __________ at near.

(RETURN TO PAGE 2 FOR ANSWER 743.)

890. resection (of the medial rectus)

891.

THE END

148. lower

149. In an upward deviating eye, the image will fall on the upper part of the retina, but the patient will interpret stimuli to this part of the retina as coming from the __________ field.

(RETURN TO PAGE 1 FOR ANSWER 149.)

297. yes

298. An ACA ratio greater than 6:1 is considered to be abnormally high.

If a subject converges 7 prism diopters for every diopter of accommodation, his ACA ratio is considered __________ than normal.

(RETURN TO PAGE 1 FOR ANSWER 298.)

446. (1) right superior rectus } either
(2) left inferior oblique } order

447. The patient in the photo is using the (1) __________ muscle and its yoke muscle, the (2) __________ .

(RETURN TO PAGE 2 FOR ANSWER 447.)

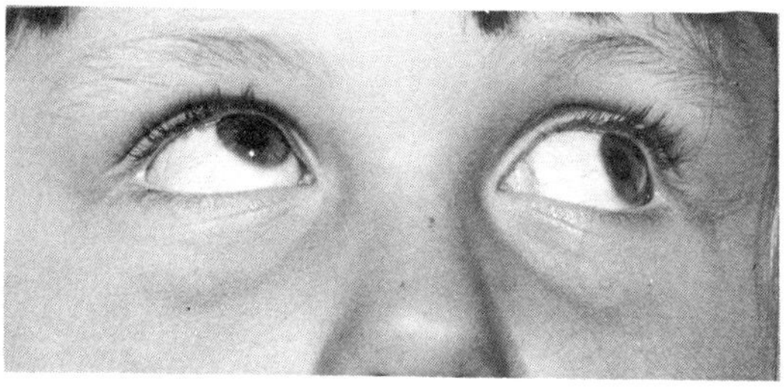

Table 1

	Squint	Amblyopes	Anisometropia of more than 2.00D	Eccentric Fixators	Vertical Primary Squints
Incidence in general population	2%	2%	2%		
Incidence in squints		50%	75%		1%
Incidence in amblyopia			50%	2%	

Index

NOTE: References in this index are to FRAME number, not to page number.